T0260852

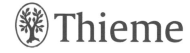

The Art of Cupping

Second Edition

Hedwig Manz
Retired Naturopathy Professional
Mainz, Germany

74 illustrations

Thieme
Stuttgart • New York • Delhi • Rio de Janeiro

Library of Congress Cataloging-in-Publication Data is available from the publisher.

This book is an authorized translation of the 6th German edition published and copyrighted 2015 by Karl F. Haug Verlag in MVS Medizinverlage Stuttgart GmbH & Co. KG, Stuttgart, Germany. Title of the German edition: Die Kunst des Schröpfens

Translator: Sabine Wilms, PhD
Langley, Washington, USA

Photographer: Peter B. Popielski, Bingen, Germany

Important note: Medicine is an ever-changing science undergoing continual development. Research and clinical experience are continually expanding our knowledge, in particular our knowledge of proper treatment and drug therapy. Insofar as this book mentions any dosage or application, readers may rest assured that the authors, editors, and publishers have made every effort to ensure that such references are in accordance with **the state of knowledge at the time of production of the book.**

Nevertheless, this does not involve, imply, or express any guarantee or responsibility on the part of the publishers in respect to any dosage instructions and forms of applications stated in the book. **Every user is requested to examine carefully** the manufacturers' leaflets accompanying each drug and to check, if necessary in consultation with a physician or specialist, whether the dosage schedules mentioned therein or the contraindications stated by the manufacturers differ from the statements made in the present book. Such examination is particularly important with drugs that are either rarely used or have been newly released on the market. Every dosage schedule or every form of application used is entirely at the user's own risk and responsibility. The authors and publishers request every user to report to the publishers any discrepancies or inaccuracies noticed. If errors in this work are found after publication, errata will be posted at www.thieme.com on the product description page.

Some of the product names, patents, and registered designs referred to in this book are in fact registered trademarks or proprietary names even though specific reference to this fact is not always made in the text. Therefore, the appearance of a name without designation as proprietary is not to be construed as a representation by the publisher that it is in the public domain.

Georg Thieme Verlag KG
Rüdigerstrasse 14, 70469 Stuttgart, Germany
+49 [0]711 8931 421, customerservice@thieme.de

Thieme Publishers New York
333 Seventh Avenue, New York, NY 10001, USA
+1-800-782-3488, customerservice@thieme.com

Thieme Publishers Delhi
A-12, Second Floor, Sector-2, Noida-201301
Uttar Pradesh, India
+91 120 45 566 00, customerservice@thieme.in

Thieme Publishers Rio
Thieme Publicações Ltda.
Edifício Rodolpho de Paoli, 25º andar
Av. Nilo Peçanha, 50 – Sala 2508
Rio de Janeiro 20020-906 Brasil
+55 21 31722297

Cover design: Thieme Publishing Group
Typesetting by Thomson Digital, India

Printed in Germany by CPI Books   5 4 3 2 1

ISBN 978-3-13-243172-0

Also available as an e-book:
eISBN 978-3-13-243173-7

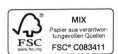

MIX
Papier aus verantwor-
tungsvollen Quellen
FSC® C083411

Contents

Part 2 Clinical Applications of Cupping Therapy

Part 3 Cupping Therapy of Indicated Disorders and Complaints

Contents

Contents

Contents

Contents

Preface

I want to remain truthful.
I want to be free from fear.
I want to have good intentions towards everybody.
Mahatma Gandhi

Cupping is a treatment modality that has been known for thousands of years. It has proven itself in popular medicine for generations and has been tested for efficacy.

The ancient method of cupping was resurrected after the end of World War II, when medications and technical therapeutic equipment were sparse. It was forgotten in times of prosperity, even though it is a safe, fast-acting treatment method, if applied correctly. Not only can it be used alone or in conjunction with other naturopathic methods, but also in combination with procedures from orthodox medicine in many cases.

We are living in a time when the number of pathogens resistant to strong antibiotics is increasing at an alarming rate. The reason for this, in the opinion of many experts, is to be found in the excessive use of these drugs, since chemical drugs must frequently be replaced with new and stronger medicines. Cupping, on the other hand, has the great advantage of being *simple* and *safe* in its application and of being effective *without drugs*.

Note

With the help of cups that attach themselves firmly to the skin by suction and cause hematomas (bruises), we can remedy functional disturbances, alleviate pain, and cure illness.

Cupping is a therapeutic technique that has become the focus of my work because of the diversity of its applications.

In our modern system of medicine, it is unfortunately still used too rarely, inspite of the fact that it offers a simple yet extremely useful treatment method—particularly in disorders related to the common cold, sinusitis, rheumatic complaints, and painful muscular tension in the back.

In addition, experientially proven cupping locations have been validated scientifically by the connections discovered between the *skin and inner organs* via the *cutivisceral* or *viscerocutaneous reflex paths*. Hence, we never treat only one organ, but *always the entire person*.

Among other treatment methods, I have been using cupping for several years. My first experiences with cupping were with my mother who normally cured my sisters and I with this technique. She advocated the view that it was better in minor illnesses to stimulate the body's self-healing than to engage "help from outside."

There are patients who simply desire a treatment method that does not involve chemical substances, medicinal side-effects, or even iatrogenic effects. Such patients prefer a therapeutic process that, when applied during illness, strengthens the organism to the point where it becomes more resistant and healthy, from illness to illness. Cupping offers all this.

Remarks about "homeopathy as concomitant therapy" complement cupping therapy. The practitioner can determine whether homeopathy promises success in any disease pattern discussed. It is understandable that I can only point to homeopathy and mention it in passing in this book. A practitioner who wants to treat effectively cannot avoid studying the technical literature on homeopathy in more detail.

I have written this book not only for the practitioners and students of naturopathy who want to be trained in cupping therapy, but also as a source of information for readers without medical training. As more than anything, the feeling of well-being in my patients after a cupping treatment has caused curiosity and raised many questions about this treatment technique, and these questions have encouraged me to explain the medical technical terms in the language of laypersons also. I thereby give them the opportunity to familiarize themselves with the entirety of this treatment method in the quiet of their home, which is something that I have found impossible to provide my patients during clinic hours due to lack of time.

I constantly hear questions like the following: What do words like extravasation, cutis, or hyperemia mean? Who besides the specialist know these terms!?

Note

For this reason, I ask practitioners to not become annoyed or impatient when I also provide the common English words for the medical technical terms and when I illustrate certain connections that would be unnecessary for professionals.

I want to explain the process and mode of action of this therapy for the layperson too in order to facilitate communication between the practitioner and the patient. Hence, I describe the harmony of the organ systems and the functional unity of the nervous system.

In my opinion, we can avoid many disappointments, errors, and misjudgments about a treatment method when we understand fully the connections between a therapy and its effect on the human body.

Although I was familiar with the effect of cupping since my childhood, I applied it with great care in my practice initially, because I was constantly reminded of the failures that this treatment method has been blamed for due to ignorance and improper application.

Now, after many years of experience, I am taking full advantage of the marvelous opportunities that cupping presents—I have yet to see any failure or mishap.

Note

This does not mean, however, that this book can replace the physician for readers without medical training, because any major or not sufficiently obvious health issue must first be evaluated by a physician or a registered complementary and alternative medicine (CAM) practitioner (Heilpraktiker).

Cupping is obviously also no substitute for necessary treatment with conventional medicine, such as surgery or antibiotics in acute illness.

It is the intention of this book to not only introduce a successful, newly rediscovered method in detail and indicate its potentials, but also its limitations, and thereby facilitate a safe application of cupping in any naturopathic clinic. Numerous photos clarify the text and thereby contribute to a deeper understanding.

I am grateful to any reader for constructive criticism. Heartfelt gratitude goes to my friend—who shall remain anonymous—for suggestions and criticism; to my daughter-in-law, Anne Popielski, for corrections and paperwork; and to all others who have contributed to the creation of this book.

Finally, my gratitude goes to everyone at Thieme Publishers for their interest and friendly cooperation in the publication of this book.

Hedwig Manz

Part 1

Introduction and Foundations

1

1 Historical Background

If you dismiss and neglect the experience of the ancients and believe that you will find the right path only in the newest treatments, you fool yourself and the people around you.

Hippocrates

The practice of cupping is over 5000 years old. The effect has remained the same; only the cups and the technique have changed over these many years. We can find the application of suction cups in the medicine of all "primitive" people, as well as in the oldest civilizations. Reports about the art of cupping were already to be found in ancient Chinese, Hindu, and Egyptian medical scriptures. The Greek physician, Hippocrates (400 BCE), who is known as the "Father of Medicine," was also very familiar with this method.

The history of medicine confirms that cupping was used successfully until the first half of the 19th century, not only in private practice but also in hospitals. In the course of the 19th century, however, great discoveries occurred that were fundamentally significant for medicine. A chemical industry developed quickly, and chemical drugs were introduced into medicine as a result of that development.

Precisely defined chemical substances aroused the interest of physicians because they had fast and specific effects. In addition, treatment was much easier with the newly discovered chemical drugs, whose mechanism of action was clearly explainable, than with the empirically based treatment methods. As a consequence, many of the old, proven treatment methods, including cupping, have gradually been forgotten in conventional Western medicine and have become the specialty of naturopaths, complementary and alternative medicine (CAM) practitioners (Heilpraktiker), and laypersons of the older generations who practiced them for self-treatment at home. Only a few physicians have continued to show interest in and research a treatment method that has survived for so many years.

In the course of centuries, cupping (especially the "bloody" variation) has unfortunately also been discredited by exaggerated and therefore often harmful applications. Publications by B. Aschner, G. Bachmann, J. Abele, A. Bier, Ch. W. Hufeland, and others confirm not only the harmful effects of cupping, which this method has long been blamed for, but also that these do not occur when it is applied correctly. These physicians also endorse the *regulating, resistance-increasing effect* of cupping and the *acceleration of recovery* in many diseases. Personally, I have also gathered a wealth of experiences with cupping throughout the years—even after critical evaluation, I have not once seen any harmful effects.

Not only in Germany, but also in many other countries, the medical trend has been reversed and therapeutic methods from complementary and alternative medicine are once again being adapted by conventional Western medicine. We owe the exploration of the ancient experience of the healing arts, which proves that we can utilize the reflex connections between the body's surface and the diseased organ, to physicians like Head and MacKenzie ("Head's zones," hyperalgesic zones), Hansen and von Staa (cutivisceral reflex paths), Scheidt (transitional segments), Pischinger (cell matrix system), and others.

The successes of alternative treatment methods can no longer be denied because they do, in fact, exist.

2 What Do We Mean by "Cupping"?

2.1 Definition and Treatment Goal

Conditions that cannot be cured with drugs are cured with iron.
Conditions that cannot be cured with iron are cured with fire. Conditions that cannot be cured with fire are incurable.

Hippocrates

Cupping refers to any natural treatment method in which *suction cups* are used in therapy.

Cupping is one of the traditional treatment methods that do not involve medicinal substances but nevertheless serve as useful weapons in the fight against many diseases or complaints. Applied correctly, the method is harmless and does not cause any adverse side-effects. The results are often fast and impressive because the body reacts within hours to cupping at the proper location.

The goal of cupping is to strengthen or activate the organism's self-healing powers, when these are not able to do so on their own. Cupping stimulates and supports the options that nature has provided the body with to resist disease.

2.2 Effects and Connections

Cupping consists of two components:
- Segmental therapy: The location of cupping is essential (see Chapter 3).
- Regulation therapy: *Extravasates* (i.e., fluid discharged from the blood vessels) act as stimuli (see Chapter 4).

Both of these components only affect the source of any illness, but not healthy body functions and tissue.

> **Note**
>
> The essential effect of cupping is the **retuning** and therefore also the regulation of disturbed body functions, as well as the alleviation of pain and cramping, improvement in blood circulation, and inhibition of inflammation.

By locally applying suction cups, *extravasates* are created and as a result of these, *hematomas* (bruises) that cause a *strong irritation*. This irritation activates the body's own localized, as well as generalized, healing powers and therefore has an *anti-inflammatory* effect, which in turn supports rapid recovery in any illness based on inflammation (e.g., pneumonia).

The process of regulating body functions *eliminates blockages* that have been caused mostly by a focal disturbance or by excessive consumption of chemical medicines, which impede the natural processes of the organism and make it ill. It is not uncommon that cupping, by eliminating blocked regulation, even brings out additional complaints, which finally indicate the location of the true disorder.

By *stimulating* circulation, cupping aims at widening the blood vessels. Increasing the blood flow at the cupping sites strengthens the metabolism and allows for faster elimination of substances that cause pain and cramping.

The above-mentioned **segmental therapy** occurs via the "Head's zones," via the so-called cutivisceral reflex paths (connections between skin and organ). Through the nervous system, this has a curative effect on disturbed *neurovegetative* functions and diseased viscera.

2.3 Methods of Application

2.3.1 Cupping Diagnosis

Cupping diagnosis allows the practitioner to determine with the aid of suction cups whether the position of the symptoms is the true location of the disease. Additionally, we can detect which organ is defective and in need of treatment.

2.3.2 "Dry" or "Bloodless" Cupping

In dry cupping, the suction cup is held over an alcohol flame in such a way that the air in it is heated. Then, the cup is placed on the treatment spot.

As the heated air cools down, it creates a vacuum inside the cup. This process sucks the skin into the cup, causing hyperemia (strong circulation) at this spot, as well as an extravasate (bloody fluid that has leaked from the vessel and is present in the tissue).

> **Note**
>
> **Cupping Massage, a Variation**
> In cupping massage, as in dry massage, a suction cup is placed on the skin, but is then moved around on the lubricated skin across a certain area. Cupping massage has a much stronger effect on blood circulation than regular massage, resulting in a large, in some places more and in other places less, pronounced extravasate in the treatment area.

2.3.3 "Wet" or "Bloody" Cupping

In wet cupping, blood is drawn at the cupping site by cutting the skin with a scarificator. The cup is placed on the skin only afterwards, to suck the blood out of the cuts. This might sound quite bloodthirsty, but in reality only involves a blood loss of 25 mL at the most. Consequently, an application of 10–15 cups of average size means losing 150–250 mL of blood.

> **Note**
>
> Wet cupping is related to bloodletting and the application of leeches. Its effect is not limited to drawing blood, but also includes a drawing out and retuning action.

2.4 Basic Therapeutic Concepts of Cupping

In spite of the fact that the cups are only placed on the skin at certain, for example, painful, parts of the body, and therefore appear to treat merely the symptoms, the aim of cupping is not all limited to suppressing the signs of the disease. Through the reflex connections, both cupping and cupping massage have a regulating and stimulating effect on the entire body and therefore a curative effect on the actual disease.

In the age of immunizations and chemically produced drugs, medical research has succeeded in controlling the great life-threatening epidemics of humankind. Nevertheless, another serious disease factor has been added: the "pharma person" (a person who takes too many drugs and uses too much medicine).

Unfortunately, strong chemical substances continue to be applied too quickly and too frequently, especially in two circumstances:

- The treatment of *functional syndromes* (an expression used in the context of disorders in which the therapist is unable to find any structural changes in the diseased organ or system and the chemical laboratory cannot contribute to the clarification of the complaints or the treatment of the patient either).
- The treatment of most types of vegetative regulation disorders, also called vegetative dystonia (the name for several symptoms that are based on disturbed regulation of the vegetative nervous system and result in a variety of functional disorders), which manifest primarily as pain at one time and as impaired circulation and insomnia at another.

To alleviate pain and to temporarily regain or feign energy and vitality, the uncontrolled reach for pills has become like a reflex movement for many people. This holds the dangers of habit and adverse drug events.

As a rule, the treatment of symptoms alone leads to chronic illness later on, which has become commonplace in our times. Cupping is not a cure-all either in my opinion. Nevertheless, the targeted application of cupping will often suffice on its own to improve a condition or guide a disturbance back to normality. In other cases, cupping can play a significant supportive role or reduce the consumption of pharmaceutical drugs, in conjunction with other proven methods and the use of effective medicines.

There is no doubt that cupping supports the natural efforts of the body, that is, the preservation or restoration of health. Additionally, it improves and complements other therapeutic methods because of its fast and reliable effects.

3 The Therapeutic Conception of Dry Cupping

3.1 Dry Cupping as Segmental Therapy

Nature heals from the inside, with the assistance of external remedies.

Thomas Aquinas

From time immemorial, almost all cultures have discovered and exploited in therapy the connections between viscera and the surface of the body. They used them to exert a healing effect on the deeper-lying organs, for example by applying warmth or cold or even by cupping. In the past, nobody knew why any of this was helpful. It simply was. It was most important to relieve complaints or achieve recovery. We are also very familiar with the influence of the skin on viscera. To reduce or eliminate pain, it is often enough to massage the corresponding skin areas lightly. The first discoveries in this field came from the Chinese. They recognized that it is possible to influence internal organs and pathologic complaints from certain points on the skin (acupuncture) or to surmise disease in certain organs on the basis of localized complaints.

3.1.1 "Head's Zones"—Reflex Paths from Skin to Organ

More recently, the British neurologist Henry Head (1861–1940) also observed this phenomenon and discovered that reflex paths exist between the body's surface (skin) and the viscera. He realized, for example, that patients with gallbladder disorders tend to be particularly sensitive to pain at the costal arches and at certain regions on the back. Kidney patients experience skin and muscle pain in the lower back on the affected side or frontally in the area around the bladder. Henry Head discovered that the *painful* and hypersensitive skin areas almost always lie on the same side of the body as the *diseased organ*. In addition, he observed that other diseases of viscera also resulted in elevated skin temperature or pain, but also disturbed blood circulation in the corresponding parts of the body's surface (often far away from the affected organ). These suggest neural interactions between the viscera and the corresponding body surface.

Head's research supplied the confirmation and therefore the scientific basis for the ancient experience of folk healing that the reflex connections from the body's surface to the diseased organ can be utilized to have a curative effect on viscera. This has been corroborated by other researchers, such as Mackenzie (myogelosis), Vogler, Krauss (osteovisceral reflex paths), Preusser, Kötschau (gelosis), Hansen and von Staa (muscle reflexes), Pischinger, Kellner, Heine, Bergsam (processes in the vegetative nervous system), and others.

The investigations of Head and other well-known scientists finally explained and proved the way in which segmental cupping therapy and cupping diagnosis work. In **segmental therapy**, the skin plays the key role. It has specific relationships to the centers of the nervous system.

The skin surface is divided into segments, so to speak, corresponding to the entrance and exit levels of the individual spinal roots in the spinal cord.

The spinal fibers pair up into spinal nerves (spinal column nerves) on the right and left between two vertebrae where they exit from the spinal cord. Since they supply strip-shaped areas of the skin, segmentation arises, which are called **segments or dermatomes**. These dermatomes are highly important also for the segmental diagnosis of spinal cord damage.

Note

In relation to the location where the nerves exit the spinal column, these segments are divided into:
   C = area of the cervical vertebrae
   T = area of the thoracic vertebrae
   L = area of the lumbar vertebrae
   S = area of the sacrum

Note

Every skin segment at the same time also has neural connections to certain viscera in the thoracic, abdominal, and sacral space. Biological functional circles (stimulatory circles) of the nervous system are in charge of the connections. These circles build a bridge between skin, central organs of the nervous system, and viscera. We now know these connections as so-called "cutivisceral/viscerocutaneous" reflex tracts (▶ Fig. 3.1).

The diseased organ sends stimuli via the vegetative nerves to the corresponding skin areas, which can respond with tension, pressure points, swelling, atrophy of connective tissue, or chronic pain. These painful, hypersensitive, or changed skin areas are referred to as **"Head's zones."**
   Each organ is represented in one zone (▶ Table 3.1).

Note

Head's zones are of practical significance for segmental therapy and diagnosis (▶ Fig. 3.2).

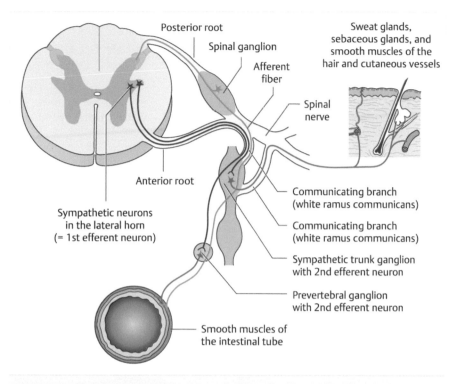

Fig. 3.1 Simplified illustration of the cutivisceral reflex paths. (From: Faller A, Schünke M. Der Körper des Menschen. 15th ed. Stuttgart: Thieme; 2008)

Table 3.1 Head's zones of the organs

Organ	Zone
Heart C3–T4	→ predominantly left
Esophagus T4–T6	→ left or right
Lungs/bronchial tubes C3–T9	→ left or right
Stomach T8–T9	→ predominantly left
Small intestine C3–T10	→ right or left
Large intestine C3–T11	→ right or left
Liver/gallbladder T8–T11	→ right
Pancreas T7–T10	→ left
Spleen T11	→ left
Kidneys/ureter T8–S4	→ left or right
Bladder on both sides T10–S4	→ left or right
Uterus/ovaries and testicles T10–L3	→ left or right

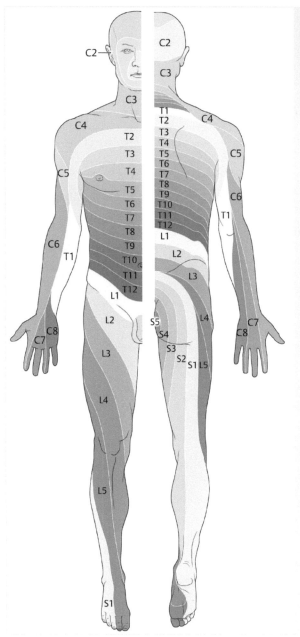

Fig. 3.2 Orienting illustration of the segments. (Schünke M, Schulte E, Schumacher U. Prometheus. THIEME Atlas of Anatomy. Head, Neck, and Neuroanatomy. Illustrations by M. Voll and K. Wesker. 3rd ed. Stuttgart: Thieme; 2020)

> **Note**
>
> **Segment reactions** almost always occur on the same side of the body as the diseased organ. Nevertheless, segments can also overlap, or the disease symptoms can, in longer-lasting illness, jump from one segment to another.

The cutivisceral and viscerocutaneous reflex paths (organ–spinal cord–skin connections) operate according to the principle of interaction or rather feedback mechanisms. In the same way that disease in the viscera manifests on the surface of the skin, we can also reversely transfer certain *skin stimuli to the viscera*.

Via these *biological functional circles*, we can on the one hand explain certain disease processes: frequent occurrence of angina pectoris episodes in cold weather for example (this path also functions in the harmful sense, e. g., sudden cooling off of the chest skin can cause a heart attack). On the other hand, we can also affect the viscera therapeutically. Among other things, we take advantage of this fact in the case of cupping therapy. By placing the cups on the skin, we address the receptors in the skin and cause not only an improved localized blood flow but also via the neural connections a more intensive blood flow in the viscera associated with the concerned skin area.

> **Note**
>
> Given the fact that cupping not only causes hyperemia, but also the formation of extravasates, the possibility of a dual therapy arises: in addition to the effect of hyperemia described above, the extravasates cause an irritation that also stimulates and accelerates the connective tissue metabolism for several days. This stimulation puts the organism in a position where it is able to restore its disturbed order through the vegetative regulatory systems.
>
> It is not uncommon that a single or only a few cupping treatments result in the complete cure of a variety of syndromes.

3.1.2 Identifying and Eliminating the Focal Disturbance

As in any type of therapy, treatment success is impossible to predetermine in cupping. In one case, a treatment will immediately have good results, but in another case that appears identical based on the symptoms, the course is completely different. This depends on each specific case of disease.

Nevertheless, cupping at the location or the segment associated with the disease is bound to fail if the true disease is located somewhere else completely. If the first treatment shows no improvement, we must consider whether there may be a distant disturbance outside the segment.

Memorize   **M!**

In such a case, we must search for the focal disturbance!
Any disease and any location of our body can turn into a focal disturbance. Any local treatment is bound to remain ineffective if we fail to eliminate the cause. This is also a necessary precondition for reducing *distant symptoms*.

On the living human body, it is not easy to visualize the segments. We have to be intimately familiar with the anatomical relationships to draw specific diagnostic conclusions on the basis of complaints that arise in the segments, which is necessary for therapy. For the quick detection of certain segments, I have found the following simplified clues helpful:

- The noticeably protruding **seventh cervical vertebra** can serve as the border between the segments **C7 and C8**.
- The **third thoracic vertebra**, which is located on the connecting line between the two shoulder ridges, can be considered as the border between the segments **T2 and T3**.
- The **seventh thoracic vertebra**, located on the lower connecting line between the two shoulder blades, can serve as the border between the segments **T6 and T7**.
- The **12th thoracic vertebra**, which can be felt as the attachment of the last rib, can be considered as the border between the segments **T11 and T12**.
- The **fourth lumbar vertebra**, located on the connecting line between the highest points of both iliac wings, can simultaneously also be considered as the border between the segments **L3 and L4**.

3.2 Dry Cupping as Regulation Therapy

Blood is a very special juice.

Goethe, Faust

When Goethe had Mephisto utter this sentence in *Faust,* he wanted to suggest that blood is a metaphor for life. This poetic image has also been fully validated from the perspective of modern science. Blood as the carrier of numerous active substances not only contributes to the management of many bodily functions but also has great diagnostic and therapeutic significance in medicine.

The therapeutic effect of blood has long been recognized. We can find theories about the way in which autohemotherapy acts on the human body in the experimental research of different physicians like Nourney, Bier, Jablonska (resistance-increasing effect), Pfeiffer (formation of antibodies), Haferkampf (summary of autohemotherapy), Hoffheinz, Petri (proteolytic ferments for resolving pneumonia), and Höveler (allergy, geriatrics, skin disorders), to name just a few.

While opinions on autohemotherapy differ, one thing is certain: autohemotherapy—**and therefore also cupping**—acts primarily in the sense of a regulation therapy.

> **Note**
>
> Regulation therapy is a naturopathic method in which a stimulus is applied to increase the organism's **power of resistance**. Alternatively—as the name of the therapy suggests—it serves to **retune disturbed self-regulatory mechanisms** of the body to enable the body to resist pathogenic influences.

The term "regulation" includes any influence that has been caused by the use of medicinal drugs or by dietetic, climatic, or even psychological measures. In general, however, regulation therapy is understood to mean the intake of substances (stimulants), primarily proteins, that have an effect on the human organism, by bypassing the gastrointestinal tract.

The most common methods with a regulating effect are *autohemotherapy, cupping,* and *autourotherapy*. Regulating substances include injections of human and animal serum (as, for example, in immunizations), blood, urine, and also boiled milk.

Autohemotherapy refers to the reinjection of small (0.1–5 mL) amounts of blood that have been drawn from the patient's vein, back into the gluteal muscles or subcutaneous tissue.

> **Note**
>
> In **cupping**, by contrast, an **extravasate** is produced by the principle of suction. The resulting **hematoma** does not disappear immediately. The enduring process or resorption lasts over several days and provokes an **increased reaction** in the tissue.

The regulating effect occurs due to the fact that the blood acts like a "foreign body" in this "foreign" environment, that is, in the soft tissue and interstitial space, and thereby has an irritating effect, which the organism tries hard to eliminate. Before the blood that has accumulated in the tissue can be removed, it must be broken down into its constituents. The disintegration of the blood in the tissue induces certain processes in the organism like the increase in antibodies—this in turn stimulates the body's defense; the blood-catabolizing agents that leak out promote the formation of new blood corpuscles and an increase of proteolytic ferments, which play a role in resolving an inflammation. This process also releases substances that stimulate the vegetative nervous system, as a result of which the blood vessels dilate and blood flow is increased. Elevated gland activity causes increased elimination, for example, of sweat, and therefore flushing of foreign substances. With these processes, the organism initiates a comprehensive therapeutic process.

3.3 Dry Cupping in the Foot Reflexology Zones

"The feet—this masterpiece—deserve our attention..."

Karin Schaffner in the poem "Der Füße Leid" (The suffering of the feet)

Just like the ears, the hands, the skull, and especially the back, the feet also have reflexology zones that originate from the neural connections between the body's inside and its surface. Through these zones, we can reflexively influence corresponding tissue structures, organs or organ systems, body functions, and body regions. Due to this fact, foot reflexology therapy can be successfully applied to cure and normalize functional disturbances, and as an accessory treatment, to improve the quality of life in patients with chronic illness. Additionally, it has been repeatedly confirmed that this procedure eases, calms, and relaxes the mind. In other words, it alleviates stress and can readily be combined with other therapies.

Memorize **M!**

The foot reflexology zones (▶ Fig. 3.3) are not identical with the Head's zones.

Foot reflexology therapy, commonly called foot reflexology massage, is rooted in the basics of zone therapy, developed by the American physician William Fitzgerald (1872–1942). As a form of therapy, it evolved over thousands of years out of traditional folk knowledge. Historical evidence exists that about 5000 years ago Native Americans, Egyptians, and Chinese already knew of the treatment of certain points and were aware that the stimulation of these points through massage, acupuncture, touching with gemstones, and cupping could have a therapeutic effect.

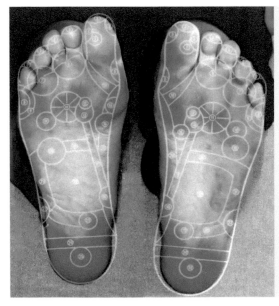

Fig. 3.3 Reflex zones on the soles of the feet.

In addition to his knowledge in conventional medicine, Fitzgerald was also familiar with traditional folk medicine. He utilized this knowledge, in combination with his discoveries of reflexive connections between internal organs and the surface of the body, to develop a system. He started out from the basic premise that the human body has 10 longitudinal zones that have corresponding reflex points on the feet and that every part of the foot can be correlated with a specific body zone. He further realized that an irritation in one of the foot reflex zones has an effect on the parts of the body or organs that are located in the associated zone of the body. In 1917, this concept and the reflexology therapy that he developed formed the foundation for modern-day foot reflexology therapy. Subsequently, these longitudinal zones were further subdivided into three cross segments each.

Foot reflexology massage was originated and developed by the physiotherapist Eunice Ingham around 1938. In Germany, it was the therapist Hanne Marquardt who applied and popularized this therapeutic method (Marquardt, 2016).

> **Note**
>
> We can thus explain the operating principle of foot reflexology by means of the neural connections between the outside and the inside of the body.

It is a unique characteristic of living organisms that they respond to stimuli. Once the stimuli are received by the organism, the nervous system processes them, whether positive or negative. During foot reflexology treatment, the stimuli, which affect and heal the organism, create neural impulses that reach the central nervous system from the periphery via neural pathways and they are processed there. Subsequently, the organs, organ systems, or parts of the body receive corresponding messages from the brain to change their functions and functional processes. In other words, these stimuli trigger reactions that cause the organism to restore normal circulation in the blood and lymph systems and to improve the elimination of metabolic end products from the organism. At the same time, they support the flow of energy to the diseased organs, activate the body's immune defenses, and strengthen its self-healing powers. In addition, we see a harmonization of the nervous system and mental state. The stimuli also contribute to the beginning or support of the healing process and, as a result, to the eventual healing of the affected organ or parts of the organism.

We can treat a number of different diseases with reflex zone therapy alone. But in most cases, it is an ideal complement to a complex therapeutic process.

Foot reflexology zones are also useful and have great practical value in the area of preventative medicine, because when a point is particularly painful or sensitive, this indicates that disturbances are present in the associated organs, organ systems, or parts of the body. A therapist who recognizes the signs from the foot reflex zones through adequate critical observation as health threats is able to prevent a potential disease, even though initially there are barely any changes visible in the associated organ (e.g., no evidence in ultrasound, X-rays, etc.).

We can see this connection between the body's surface and inside reflected in the fact that it is not only an organ itself that is affected in case of a disease but also the surrounding subcutaneous and connective tissues. When palpating a diseased person, this frequently manifests in specific areas of the body as poor blood circulation, sensitivity to touch or pressure, or swelling or even deposits or knots in the connective tissue (myogeloses (Abele, 2005)).

Memorize   M!

Foot reflexology therapy is generally appropriate for all people, from infants to the elderly, because age presents neither an obstacle nor a contraindication.

Contraindications for foot reflexology therapy are:
• Venous and arterial inflammation in the legs and feet.
• Pregnancy: high-risk pregnancy.
• Acute cardiac insufficiency.
• Acute circulatory problems.
• Diseases on the feet that make treatment impossible.

It is, however, entirely appropriate to treat tumor patients. While foot reflexology therapy will not cure the disease, it can improve a number of attendant symptoms considerably.

No standardized illustrations of the foot reflex zones exist, only a number of mutually divergent ones. Nevertheless, experience has shown that the small area of the reflex zones on the sole and back of the foot does in fact reflect the entirety of the body with all its organs, muscle groups, and parts, and that it is possible to influence specific regions of the body reflexively by treating corresponding zones. This experience has remained consistent through the centuries, regardless of variations in the depictions of reflex zones.

Note

We can affect the left half of the body through the left foot, and the right half through the right foot. The reflex zones for the internal organs are located on the soles of the feet, and the sides of the feet are in charge of the bones, joints, and spinal column.

The most popular reflex zone, which is located in the middle of the soles of the feet, is the so-called "network of the sun," or in other words, the solar plexus. It is the most significant center that exerts control over the most important internal organs of the human body. It plays an important role in steering the various bodily functions and emotions. Traditional Chinese medicine was well aware of the reason why it considered the solar plexus to be of central importance. By treating this zone, the practitioner has access to a balancing intervention, in order to alleviate complaints, affect illnesses positively, and bring the body and soul back from disharmony to harmony. For this reason, applying cups in this location is not only recommended for the treatment of different illnesses but also for the sake their prevention.

As already mentioned above, in traditional Chinese medicine the corresponding foot reflex zones are also stimulated by means of cupping. Applying cups has the advantage that the practitioner does not get tired, as is often the case with massages. And yet, dry cupping of the foot reflex zones does not make traditional reflex zone massage expendable; it is still indispensable. Cupping on the foot reflex zones should be viewed as a therapeutic alternative to foot massage.

Because the skin of the feet tends to be dry, it is recommended to rub lotion or oil on them before cupping.

Memorize   **M!**

If the stimulation caused by cupping is experienced as very painful (which can happen very rarely, at the beginning of a treatment), remove the cup. This pain is an indication of the patient's tolerance limit. Wait until the next treatment session before trying again to stimulate this reflex zone. Tolerable pain that does not exceed the patient's pain tolerance limit never have to be a reason to stop the treatment. Nevertheless, the length of cupping can be informed by this. As a general rule, a cupping treatment on the soles of the feet takes 10–20 minutes.

3.4 The Effects of Dry Cupping on the Human Body

The physician has only one task, to heal, and if he succeeds in this, it is irrelevant how he succeeded in it!

Hippocrates

The effects of cupping therapy are varied. You can often recognize it by a pleasant fatigue that occurs immediately after cupping. Hence, you should not deny the patient a potentially therapeutic sleeplike rest afterwards to allow the possibility of far-reaching regulating processes to take effect.

Note

The regulating effect of cupping manifests in patients in a *renewed responsiveness to therapies* that had previously become ineffective. We can also observe *increased resistance* against infectious diseases.

Note

Cupping therapy stimulates the body's defense in general, as a result of which inflammations are stopped or prevented. The healing of many diseases is clearly accelerated or the complaints are at least alleviated.

Most visible are the effects of cupping in:
• Acute and subacute bronchitis.
• Angina.
• Influenza.
• Pneumonia.
• Major common colds.

A cupping treatment applied on the first or second day brings substantial improvement for the patient in a short time, and recovery can be observed almost immediately. The healing process is smooth and without complications common in treatment with medicinal drugs.

Even in cases where the patient comes for treatment only in the *delayed stage,* cupping therapy is recommended for fast recovery and prevention of secondary complications. Grogginess disappears quickly in difficult cases, and you will notice an increase in the will to recover and in vital energy.

> **Note**
>
> There is no other disease where the therapist succeeds as quickly as in diseases of the *respiratory organs.* Hence, these are the true domain of cupping.
>
> In addition, disorders of the *digestive tract, kidneys,* or *urinary tracts,* as well as *cardiovascular diseases* also respond well to cupping therapy.
>
> *Chronic diseases* that manifest in different forms and locations are a difficult, but also rewarding field for cupping therapy.

I often observe a surprisingly rapid pain-relieving effect, especially in several conditions where all other measures have failed. **Persistent pain** in the area of the *spinal column*, in *neuralgia, in chronic rheumatoid arthritis*, as well as in *headaches* that were caused by muscle tensions can generally be affected quite well.

When applied at the right locations, cupping relaxes the muscles, widens the blood vessels, and stimulates circulation. This allows for a faster elimination of pain-causing substances, as a result of which pain is reduced.

Similarly, essential nutrients are transported more rapidly to the location of the disorder by the increased circulation. This encourages the natural healing process.

Patients who had been taking strong analgesic drugs for years became almost pain-free or at least able to greatly reduce the amount of pain killers they were taking after a few cupping treatments. Patients suffering from insomnia were finally able to sleep well or at least better after treatment.

Again and again, we are surprised by the improvement in subjective general health in most patients, often manifesting already after a single treatment. As I observed in many cases in my practice, patients feel substantially fresher and more productive.

> **Note**
>
> A great advantage of cupping therapy is the fact that it can be combined with other therapies and that patients require neither bed rest nor any other special care in the course of treatment. During this time, they are able to pursue their jobs and any other activities.
>
> **Nevertheless:** While cupping therapy does not cause any harm, it must still not be applied uncritically or indiscriminately because of this. Every case requires a *precise indication* in the treatment with cupping.

4 Self-regulatory Mechanisms in the Body— A Crash Course for Patients

4.1 The Harmony of the Organ Systems

Observe how the things in the world are made, and differentiate between the forces acting on them and the goal.

Marc Aurelius

The body and its functions are two basic aspects of life that cannot be separated from each other. The human body develops meaningfully in growth and metabolism. Its internal unity makes possible its astounding organization and unimaginable regulatory abilities, on the basis of which it succeeds in continuously adjusting to new circumstances.

To better recognize the effects of cupping, understanding the basic structure of the organ systems and the functional processes in the human body is indispensable.

The human body is constructed of cells, tissues, organs, and organ systems. In accordance with their location, structure, and functions, the individual organs and organ systems vary considerably. Nevertheless, the human organism is more than just a sum of its organs. It is an *integrated whole* that cannot be separated.

The uniqueness of humans is not found in the details of our bodily structure, but in the functional harmony of the organs and organ systems, which guarantees the continuous, mutually interdependent, frictionless completion of all life processes.

The body consists of billions of cells, which are the smallest building blocks with vital properties, only visible under a microscope. These guarantee internal unity. Depending on their specialization, the cells exhibit very different shapes and functions (e.g., muscle cells, blood corpuscles, neurons, etc.).

Cells that are structured similarly in view of one or several similar functions form associations for certain tasks, namely tissue (e.g., muscle tissue, glandular tissue, nerve tissue, etc.).

Tissues in turn combine by practical associations and in abundant combinations to form organs that are charged with performing certain functions. Tissues and organs combine into systems in which the links are formed by functional complexes, such as digestion, respiration, and so on. All cells for the construction of organs are held together and connected to each other by intercellular fluid.

Nerve tracts and hair blood vessels (capillaries) end freely in the intercellular fluid without having direct cell contact. The intercellular fluid, also called tissue fluid, facilitates microcirculation and thereby the completion of all vital processes. This functional unity of cells, nerves, capillaries, and tissue fluid, called "**vegetative ground system**" by the researcher A. Pischinger, constitutes *an impulse-transmitting system of information in the* organism. As a result, every cell in the body is constantly linked indirectly with every other healthy cell. Only cells damaged by irritation, that is, diseased cells, are shut out of this comprehensive information system. Hence, they create a gap in the functional unity and thereby limit organ activity.

The human skeleton determines the shape and form of the body: Its hard and resistant components are the bones and cartilage. Our body is constructed with the purpose of moving it.

4.1.1 Locomotor System

The locomotor system, consisting of muscles and the skeleton, fulfills the task of movement. The framework of the bones is moved in the joints by the muscles. Muscle activities are coordinated through the nervous system. Blood and lymph nourish the locomotor system.

As humans, we express our emotional state with facial muscles and hand movements. Muscle movements allow us to communicate thoughts to others in speaking and writing. Movements facilitate the execution of all other functions that are connected to human life (e.g., changes in location, mechanical influence on the environment).

The body must not only preserve itself and expand by growth, it also needs energy to maintain a stable body temperature and perform chemical and mechanical tasks. This energy has to be supplied to the body through food. The foodstuffs that we absorb by eating are ultimately supposed to reach the individual cells of the organism to guarantee their work. To make this happen, food must be broken down into its chemical components to the point where these become water-soluble. Only then can they penetrate the intestinal wall to enter the blood and be transported to the cells of the organs.

4.1.2 Digestive System

The digestive system has the task of taking the ingested food and breaking it up, liquefying it, and making it absorbable by means of ferments and enzymes. We consider the digestive system to include the oral cavity, the middle and lower sections of the throat, the esophagus, the stomach, the small intestine, the liver and pancreas, the large intestine, the rectum, and the anus.

The nutrients that have been absorbed into the body, for their part, cannot be transformed into energy by the cells without outside assistance. For this process, the body needs oxygen.

4.1.3 Respiratory System

The respiratory system facilitates breathing. By means of our respiratory organs, we inhale the oxygen in the air and exhale carbon dioxide and water vapor. Respiration leads to a step-by-step combustion of carbon and hydrogen, with the help of oxygen. This is a process that supplies energy and is essential for life.

We refer to the gas exchange between the pulmonary alveoli and capillaries of the lung on the one hand and the atmosphere on the other as external respiration. Tissue, or internal, breathing describes the process by which the blood conveys oxygen to the tissue and in its place takes in carbon that has accumulated there. The respiratory passages include the nasal cavity and the upper and middle section of the throat, the larynx, the trachea, the bronchial tubes, and the lungs.

To ensure the constant supply of blood to all parts of the organism, a separate transportation system is necessary.

4.1.4 Circulatory System

The circulatory system consists of blood vessels of different sizes and structures that are in charge of bringing blood into the immediate vicinity of all cells. The heart is the motor of this cycle. It pumps blood that has been replenished with oxygen into the large arteries of the body and pumps used blood that flows in from the large veins of the body back into the lungs.

Blood is one large transport organ that transports nutritive and constructive substances as well as hormones and other active agents to the individual organs and tissues.

The organ systems described here supply the working cell groups of the body with energy-supplying substances and with oxygen. Nevertheless, tissue activity also leads to the formation of substances that the body has no more use for. These must be discharged. The main organs of discharge are the kidneys.

4.1.5 Urinary System

The urinary system performs the vital functions of discharge, especially of substances produced during protein metabolism, but also of water and salts as well as foreign matter, medicinal and recreational drugs, and so on. The urinary system also has the ability to regulate body fluid. It is comprised of the two kidneys, the two ureters, the bladder, and the urethra.

4.1.6 Reproductive Organs

In the human body, its functions also include reproductive capacity. The reproductive organs do not serve the preservation of the body, but the preservation of the species. Their activity produces a new living being of the same genus.

To be able to survive, the human organism must defend itself against a wide variety of pathogens, against extraneous substances of all types (proteins, toxins, etc.), as well as against diseased cells.

4.1.7 Immune System

The immune system enables the organism to recognize and destroy substances that are foreign to the body or have become so. It can be divided into two systems: the *humoral* (i.e., settled in the bodily fluids) and the *cellular* (i.e., settled in the cells) immune systems work together and are inseparable because the cells construct the antibodies, and all antibodies in the blood originate in the cells. The cellular immune system is superior to the humoral immune system and directs it.

In addition, the body also contains organs that regulate its relationship with the environment: the sensory organs. These are perceptive organs that are directed toward specific impulses.

4.1.8 Sensory Organs

With special receptors, the sensory organs receive messages (impulses) from the outside and transmit these via neural pathways to the neural central agencies: the brain and the spinal cord.

In humans, we distinguish between the sense of smell, taste, vision, hearing, position, touch, temperature, and balance.

Nature has made ample provisions in the structure of the human body to ensure the harmony of the organ systems as a whole, as well as the equal distribution of individual body functions, thereby creating the necessary balance of all activities for the whole organism. At one point, organs or organ systems must be stimulated to increase their activity; at another point, they must be slowed down in their activity.

4.1.9 Hormonal Control System

For coordinating activities, the human body has two control systems: the hormonal and nervous systems.

The hormonal control system facilitates chemical control by means of certain active substances, namely hormones. The endocrine glands produce the hormones, which circulate around the body in the blood circulatory pathways as the distribution system. Hormones are substances that do not themselves participate in cell metabolism but are able to regulate tissue activity by their presence. Their effects are slow and directly aimed at the activity of specific organs and tissue.

4.1.10 Nervous System

Consisting of the central and the vegetative nervous system, the nervous system operates through nervous impulses that permit a rapid and exact transfer of information. Both the hormonal and nervous systems operate in mutual dependence. The hormones influence the nervous system, and all endocrine glands are amply supplied with vegetative nerves.

Depending on the particular circumstances, pathogenic irritations result either in defense, in adaptation to the changed situation, or in compensating for misdirected or inhibited reactions. Harmful irritations that can no longer be balanced out by the complicated control system cause entire regulatory systems of the organism to become blocked and result in disturbed tissue and organ functions, that is, to disease.

While a disorder primarily manifests in an organ, it in affects more or less the entire organism, based on the body's structure and functions.

4.2 Focal Disturbance as Regulatory Blockage in the Body

As long as we allow the true cause of a disorder to persist, all therapeutic methods are only a drop in the bucket.

Prof. H. Much

The organism's regulatory capacity can be blocked by a certain type of disease that we refer to as focal disturbance.

> **Note**
>
> We regard as focal disturbance any location of the body that has changed pathologically and has acquired the ability to cause or preserve disorders elsewhere beyond its closest vicinity.

The most common focal disturbances are found in the head area, for example, in the periodontal and maxillary area and at the tonsils. The sinuses and internal organs like the liver, gallbladder, and intestines can also assume characteristics of a focal disturbance, whether bacteria have settled there or not. Finally, we can consider chronic stress situations as focal disturbance because they deplete the organism's power of resistance.

> **Note**
>
> Focal disturbances can impact health by different processes, most notably by irritating the surrounding nerves that are disturbed in turn and then convey misinformation to the rest of the nervous system.

A focal disturbance can, however, also lie dormant for years, as a result of which the health of the rest of the organism is spared damage by the disturbance for a long time, while the body is able to isolate the disturbance locally. However, this can severely weaken the body's defense. As a result, the body is much more susceptible to other diseases.

Since the focal disturbance is anchored in the vegetative ground system as misinformation, it is also possible that it can suddenly be activated without any visible cause or by infection or trauma (also due to surgery). This will then result in unimpeded distal effects in the rest of the organism. Chronic tonsillitis, for example, remains a local disease in one patient, but causes strain as a focal disturbance on other organs in another.

Focal disturbances can trigger or cause any type of internal disorder, or even prevent recovery from other diseases. They are quite malicious and difficult to find because they do not cause symptoms typical for the disturbance, but result merely in limited functionality in other organs or even just pain in other locations. Thus, right-sided headache, for example, points to a chronically impaired gallbladder, and the sinuses can be responsible for the occurrence of acute sciatic pain.

The existence of a focal disturbance is usually first indicated by functional disorders in which the lack of clinically measurable pathological findings often suggests a psychosomatic background that tends to be treated with psychotropic drugs.

The following can indicate the existence of a focal disturbance:

- Pain that fails to respond to locally applied therapy.
- Occurrence of additional complaints after cupping.
- Sudden occurrence of an illness after trauma. It is only after this additional strain that the local isolation of the damaging effects of a focal disturbance breaks down.
- Fatigue, sleep disorders, sensitivity to changes in weather.
- Normal laboratory results in spite of existing illness.

In such cases, we must consider a distal disturbance, look for the focus, and treat correspondingly.

A disease that is caused by a focal disturbance can only be improved or cured by treating the focal disturbance. Therapy at the site of the symptoms may bring some relief, but only temporarily. My daily practice has proven over and over that a symptomatic treatment does not bring lasting cure.

Additional factors that can lead to a **regulatory blockage of the organism** are many medicinal drugs such as *psychotropic drugs, corticoids, antibiotics, antiallergics,* and so on.

Long-standing dysregulation, whether caused by a focal disturbance or medication, are also responsible for making the human organism inaccessible to therapy. It is only by regulation therapies such as cupping that we can break through the regulatory blockage and then make treatment possible.

By describing regulatory blockage as mentioned before, I want to stress once again that the occurrence of additional complaints after cupping is to be regarded not as the harmful effect of cupping but as the body's natural reaction. The body signals in this way that a focal disturbance is present.

The formation and existence of so-called regulatory blockages in the human body due to the factors mentioned above have been scientifically proven by Rost with thermography and by Pischinger and Kellner with iodometry.

4.3 The Functional Unity of the Nervous System

The nervous system can be compared to a telephone network, which facilitates the rapid and immediate contact of separate locations to each other and therefore a "remote control."

Prof. Dr. Lucas

The whole reaction of the nervous system should be regarded as a functional unity. At the foundation of nerve activity, a large number of stimulatory cycles (functional cycles, ▶ Fig. 4.1) are in charge of transferring stimuli and impulses, which they do by means of feedback mechanisms. Within a stimulatory cycle, we distinguish the following:

Receiver (receptor) → adducting line → center with switchboard → abducting line → executing organ (e.g., muscles).

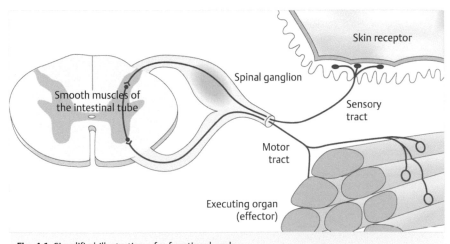

Fig. 4.1 Simplified illustration of a functional cycle.

The maintenance and continuation of life is to a large degree dependent on the ordered mode of operation of the nervous system.

The entire nervous system is divided into two separate systems: the central and peripheral nervous system or the cerebrospinal nervous system and the vegetative nervous system.

The division of the nervous system has more theoretical than practical significance. Both systems are intimately connected with each other. The nerve tracts are never more than opposing sides of stimulatory cycles. Both systems have neural centers and peripheral nerves.

The brain and spinal cord are the central organs for both of these systems. Together, they are regarded as the central or cerebrospinal nervous system.

The nerves of the brain and spinal cord innervate the head, trunk, and extremities and thereby also form the peripheral part of the nervous system.

The **vegetative nervous system** innervates particularly the bowels and regulates respiration, circulation, digestion, metabolism, secretion, and excretion, as well as reproduction.

The performance of the nervous system is related to the ability to perceive, transmit, and process impulses. The nervous system is constructed in accordance with these abilities. Sensory cells are developed for **impulse perception**; the nerves are developed for **impulse transmission**; and the brain and spinal cord are developed for **impulse processing.**

Both the central and vegetative nervous systems are composed of nerve cells and their extensions. These are the nutritive structural units in the nerve tissue. A nerve cell with the total of its extensions is referred to as neuron. The usually short, branching extensions, which receive impulses from other nerve cells are known as dendrites. The usually long extensions that transmit the impulse away from the cell are called axons (▶ Fig. 4.2). Their length can be up to 1 m in adults.

In both systems, the peripheral nerves consist of axons of nerve cells, which are bundled by connective tissue into larger cables.

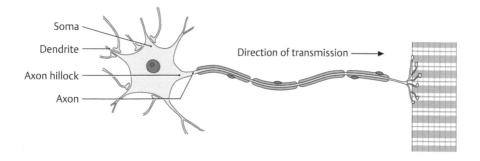

Fig. 4.2 Simplified illustration of a nerve cell. (From: Duale Reihe Anatomie. 2nd ed. Stuttgart: Thieme; 2010)

4.3.1 The Cerebrospinal Nervous System

Also called **central** or **somatic nervous system**, the cerebrospinal nervous system regulates the relationship with the environment, transmits perceptions as well as movement, and can be influenced intentionally. Environmental stimuli that act on the body are transmitted by the sensory cells via sensory nerves to the central nervous system. The central nervous system responds to the stimulus with an order that is transmitted to the muscles via the motor nerves. The organism, however, not only responds to the environment, but also affects it. This scenario again results in a corresponding functional cycle.

The **brain** is the starting point for 12 so-called *brain nerve pairs*. These pairs are numbered with Roman numerals according to the order in which they exit the brain. The brain nerves run directly from the brain to the face, mouth, and throat. Only the tenth brain nerve (the cranial nerve X, the vagus nerve) runs all the way down to the intestinal tract.

The spinal cord is the starting point for 31 pairs of spinal cord nerves, also called spinal nerves. Each spinal cord nerve has two roots on the side of the spinal cord: a dorsal root (motor) and a ventral root (sensory). The roots combine inside the vertebral column into spinal cord nerves and leave the vertebral column in pairs to the left and right between two vertebrae.

At the level of the dorsal root, we find a spinal ganglion, which contains the sensory neurons of the central nervous system and the vegetative nervous system.

The **spinal cord nerves** are differentiated according to the point where they emerge from the spinal cord (▶ Fig. 4.3):

- Eight pairs of **cervical (i.e., neck) nerves**, corresponding to segments **C1–C8**. These are the origin for the nerves of the upper limbs, but also for the **phrenic nerve.**
- Twelve paired **thoracic (i.e., chest) nerves**, corresponding to segments **T1–T12**. They supply the costal musculature.
- Five paired **lumbar nerves**, corresponding to segments **L1–L5**. They innervate the legs.
- Five paired **sacral nerves**, corresponding to segments **S1–S5**.
- One pair of **coccygeal nerves—Co1**.
- The lowest nerves fuse to form the **sciatic nerve**, which runs through the buttocks and thighs into the feet.

The segmental nerves partly combine into networks before they run to the effector organs. Among the most important networks are the neck, arm, and lumbosacral networks.

The spinal cord and brain nerves form the **peripheral nervous system**. Its primary function is to transmit impulses from the periphery, for example, the skin and muscles of the limbs, to the central nervous system on the one hand, and from the central nervous system to the muscles of the limbs on the other. The nerves that run from the periphery (from the skin) to the center are called **impulse-transmitting (afferent) or sensory nerves**.

The nerves that run from the center (from the spinal cord or brain) to the executing organs are **called motion-triggering (efferent) or motor nerves**. The motor nerves innervate the muscles.

The sensory nerves innervate the skin. All organs are innervated by **viscerosensory nerves**, while the smooth muscles of the bowels are innervated by **visceromotor nerves**.

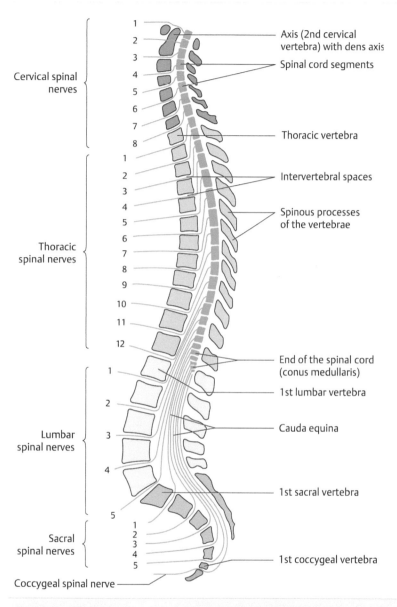

Cervical spinal nerves

Thoracic spinal nerves

Lumbar spinal nerves

Sacral spinal nerves

Coccygeal spinal nerve

Axis (2nd cervical vertebra) with dens axis

Spinal cord segments

Thoracic vertebra

Intervertebral spaces

Spinous processes of the vertebrae

End of the spinal cord (conus medullaris)

1st lumbar vertebra

Cauda equina

1st sacral vertebra

1st coccygeal vertebra

Fig. 4.3 Simplified illustration of the spinal cord and the exiting spinal cord nerves. (From: Faller A, Schünke M. Der Körper des Menschen. 15th ed. Stuttgart: Thieme; 2008)

4.3.2 The Vegetative Nervous System

Also called autonomic, involuntary, or vital nervous system, the vegetative nervous system regulates all important vital functions, such as respiration, circulation, digestion, hunger and thirst, and so on. It innervates the internal organs, the blood vessels, and the sweat glands in the skin. The neurons and axons of the vegetative nervous system are found in all parts of the body.

The vegetative nervous system operates without being directly influenced by the mind. Nevertheless, its performance is closely linked with that of the central and peripheral nervous systems.

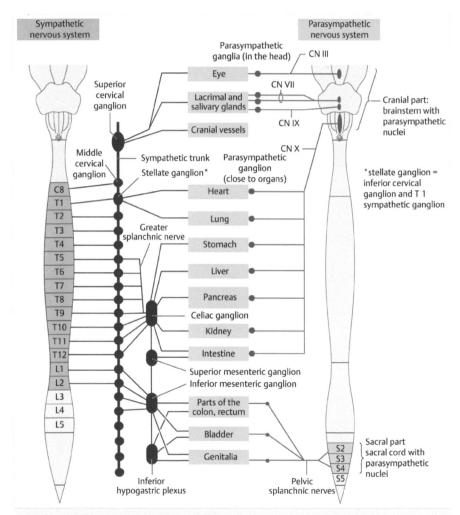

Fig. 4.4 Simplified illustration of the vegetative nervous system. (Schünke M, Schulte E, Schumacher U. THIEME Atlas of Anatomy. Head, Neck, and Neuroanatomy. Illustrations by M. Voll and K. Wesker. 3rd ed. Stuttgart: Thieme; 2020)

To ensure the harmonious activity of the internal organs, the vegetative nervous system is divided into a sympathetic part and a parasympathetic part. From a functional perspective, these operate as antagonists. In healthy persons, however, neither of these parts has complete dominance over the other. All organs that are influenced by the vegetative nervous system are supplied with sympathetic and parasympathetic nerve fibers (▶ Fig. 4.4).

The Sympathetic Nervous System

The sympathetic nervous system is comprised of nerve fibers that emerge from the spinal cord at the level of the thoracic and lumbar vertebrae. These run through ganglia, which are lined up on both sides of the spinal column into the chain-like sympathetic trunk, to the internal organs and blood vessels. With the exception of the cervical and lumbar sections, there are as many ganglia as there are segmental nerves. The sympathetic nervous system is set up for momentary maximum performance: It accelerates the heart beat and respiration, increases blood pressure, widens the coronary arteries and bronchial tubes, etc.

The Parasympathetic Nervous System

The parasympathetic nervous system consists of nerve fibers of the vagus nerve, which originates in the brain. Other parts of the parasympathetic nervous system originate in the spinal cord. The parasympathetic nervous system serves the purpose of rest, that is, slowdown of different body functions, for example, heart rate and respiration, constriction of the pupils or coronary arteries and bronchial tubes, and so on.

In spite of this division into central and vegetative nervous system, which is primarily of theoretical significance, both systems are intimately linked together. It is only as a whole that they facilitate and regulate the activities of the organism.

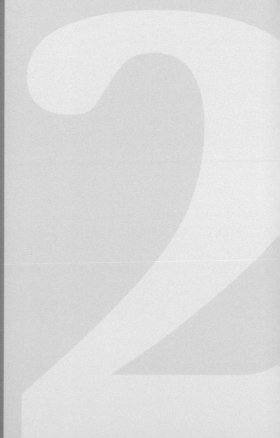

Part 2

Clinical Applications of Cupping Therapy

5 Preliminary Comments

Cupping is a therapeutic method that strengthens the body's healing power rather than drowning it in the chemical substances of medications. It does not take away the organism's ability to heal itself and does not annihilate nature's healing power. This is a healing art whose quality is reflected in the fact that its effectiveness has persisted for 5000 years already.

"The art of cupping" consists of the multiplicity of options we have for influencing the whole body. The therapist not only treats by means of suction cups and strengthens the body's resistance against disease, but also makes a diagnosis.

Just as in any other art, though, those who want to apply the "art of cupping" must first master its techniques and acquire a certain amount of knowledge. When skillfully administered, cupping can certainly be seen as an extension and enrichment of our modern medicine.

We attempt to explore all possibilities that this therapy offers, as long as they are reasonable and responsible. Cupping on its own often suffices to improve a disease or to cure. Of course, there are also cases where cupping only plays a supporting but essential role alongside other proven methods.

Cupping by nature focuses on *infectious and functional diseases.* While we cannot cure organic changes with cupping, we can at least improve the functional disturbances that are caused by diseased organs.

This book gives instructions for indications and therapies. Of course, the discussions can only contain tips because there are just as many disorders as there are patients. This book can therefore not lay claim to completeness.

All therapists know that no two cases of disease are alike and that cupping cannot be a cure-all method. When administering cupping, we must always adapt to the circumstances, not overvalue our successes, and remain critical. This is the necessary precondition for evaluating cupping according to the principle: *Primum nil nocere,* meaning: First, do no harm!

6 Dry Cupping

6.1 Cupping Diagnostics

6.1.1 Fundamentals

Before the therapy, the gods have placed the diagnosis... But any diagnosis remains idle talk, as long as it does not help therapeutically.

Volhard

The human body possesses a warning signal system, which responds to functional disturbances or dangerous influences on the organism by sending warning signals, called signs of disease or symptoms. This warning signal system is directed by the nervous system. The warning signals first reach specific switch and control centers, which mobilize the body's own resistance.

Memorize	M!
Fever, pain, a sensation of pressure at certain locations of the body, dizziness, and so on, for example, are not diseases but signals of an internal defense reaction in the body on the one hand, and signs of disease that alert us that there is something wrong with our body on the other.	

Fever and pain are not the only signs that indicate when something is out of order inside us. The skin, eyes, mouth, tongue, hair, and nails also reveal much information about disturbances of the internal organs, if we are able to read certain signs correctly.

The ability to recognize disease on the basis of external signs is as old as medicine itself. For the therapist, easily recognizable changes that occur parallel to the symptoms of a disorder are of great help in diagnosis. They notify us that the body's regulatory mechanisms are overburdened.

These external signs may appear, but they don't have to. The intensity of external body reactions also differs from person to person; it can be strong at certain times and change during the course of the disease.

The development of laboratory and high-tech medicine has caused diagnosis on the basis of external signs to become less and less important, in spite of the fact that external phenomena are very useful in the early identification of disease—they can precede the outbreak of internal disorders by a long time.

External disease signs were more or less well known to practitioners in antiquity for diagnostic purposes, but have increasingly fallen into oblivion as technology has been introduced into modern medicine. They have, however, been preserved in naturopathy and thereby been rescued into the present.

This is important because, even in the age of computerized medicine, technology is not able to predict everything about our vital processes, and the body continues to express its suffering in the same way as before. We must take note of this!

Diagnosis in the traditional sense refers to the identification of disease on the basis of the sum of all symptoms and the results of a variety of specific technological and chemical tests.

Naturopathy, on the other hand, is continuously accused of administering treatments uncritically and without sufficient clinical clarification. Here, we must stress emphatically that people who resort to naturopathic therapies are mostly chronically ill patients. Such patients have long since endured clinical diagnosis and the resulting therapies without hoped-for results.

Nevertheless, what troubles patients and therapists most are not the clearly diagnosable diseases, but the "**functional disturbances**" that the majority of patients suffer from. Not even the latest diagnostic methods are able to identify clearly functional disturbances that manifest in numerous varied syndromes, and are all too often dismissed as psychosomatic disorders. As a result of this, out-of-hospital diagnostic options can and should be utilized.

We naturopaths are not satisfied with the results of clinical tests alone. We first make a diagnosis on the basis of a detailed patient history. For this purpose, we trace the succession of all illnesses of a patient beginning with birth, but pay particular attention to those that could be a cause of the present disorder. In addition, our diagnosis is based on careful observation of the patient as well as an extensive *physical examination*. This also includes special naturopathic diagnostic procedures that allow us to identify the disease cause before we initiate treatment.

This is significant because naturopathy believes that finding and eliminating the cause is the essential precondition for curing.

Diagnosis is a very important, but also very difficult aspect of medicine. At least for the layperson, it is not easy to attribute observed complaints or skin changes correctly to specific diseases.

In spite of all the accuracy of traditional diagnosis, it is often also no more than a preliminary tool for the therapist. We learn in clinic that a focal disturbance can be present in the body, which sends out distant disturbances and quite frequently points to another disease.

Not many people are aware that **suction cups are also a tool that can serve diagnostic purposes**. Unfortunately, this is an art that is practiced all too rarely but is easy to learn and meaningful and rewarding.

6.1.2 Symptoms: Hyperemia and Extravasation at the Cupping Sites

Cupping can greatly facilitate the search for the true locus—not of all, but of many disturbances.

It is only after we have applied the cups that we can determine with absolute accuracy whether the pathogenic disturbance that requires treatment is truly present at the cupping site or not. The reason for this is as follows:

> **Note**
>
> Sites where **extravasates** form after cupping must always be regarded as **localization** of the disease or as **remote irritation** of the segment belonging to the diseased organ.

Extravasates never form at healthy locations, but only at diseased places or at Head's zones associated with a diseased organ. The reason for this is an extremely complex inflammatory process that I can explain here only briefly.

The inflammation originates as a defense reaction of the organism and its tissue against a variety of harmful attacks of all kinds (pathogens and their toxins, foreign substances, etc.). The inflammation is generally intended to prevent and eliminate the harmful attacks and their effects on the organism.

Four symptoms mark the inflammatory process:
- Hyperemia (redness).
- Swelling.
- Pain.
- Reduced functionality.

The **redness** results from a localized dilation of blood vessels, a process in which the increased influx of blood to the diseased location simultaneously makes the location appear warmer. The **swelling** is caused by a secretion of white blood corpuscles from the blood vessels by an accumulation of tissue fluid. The pressure of this accumulation on the fine nerve endings causes **pain**. The swelling and pain together bring about the **reduced functionality**. At the site of the inflammation, biochemical and physiochemical changes occur that result in permanent circulatory disturbances with increased tissue permeability for blood plasma and blood cells.

It is precisely this increased permeability of the tissue that is utilized in cupping therapy:

> **Note**
>
> As a result of the vacuum created in the suction cup, the **blood only issues from diseased locations** or Head's zones of diseased organs, never from healthy ones.

6.1.3 Complex of Symptoms: Increase in Local Blood Circulation and Paleness of the Skin

> **Note**
>
> In addition to the occurring **hyperemia** and **extravasates** at the cupping site, a conspicuous localized **paleness of the skin** is also of significance for diagnosis.

Under normal circumstances, the skin turns red in the vicinity of the applied suction cup. Paleness of skin there, by contrast, indicates a lack of circulation in a certain area of tissue. Acute or chronic lack of circulation can have different causes and effects on organs or parts of the organism. As a rule, blood circulation supplies every organ with the appropriate amount of blood for its requirements. Reduced circulation (**ischemia**), however, can only appear if the blood supply via the arteries or the backflow of blood via the veins is impeded. Several causes should be considered:
- Inflammatory or degenerative **tissue change.**
- **Thrombosis.**
- **Embolism.**
- **Vascular spasms.**
- **Constricted lumen** due to pathological processes in the vicinity.

> **Note**
>
> The most common cause of ischemia is **localized chronic muscle tension**, which can also trigger arterial spasms.

Ischemia due to muscular hypertonicity in the neck, for example, can in turn trigger many other conditions like: *headache*, nightly *paresis* (a type of numbness) in the upper extremities as well as *pain* in the *shoulders*, in the *elbow*, and in the *back*.

6.1.4 Therapeutic Success as Diagnostic Evidence

> **Note**
>
> A diagnosis can also be deduced from the success of cupping.

For example, placing a suction cup in the area of the sciatic nerve in cases with suspected sciatic pain can often bring relief from complaints or absence of sciatic symptoms.

The treatment will, however, be ineffective if the pain has other causes.

Reluctant Improvement of Existing Complaints

<table>
<tr><td>

Note

Reluctant improvement of existing complaints **(mostly in long-lasting disease, e.g., joint pain)** also confirms a correct diagnosis.

</td></tr>
</table>

These effects of cupping suggest that the cups were placed on the correct, that is, the diseased, location. It is important for diagnosis that the resulting improvement persists. If this is the case, you should continue treatment at the same place until you have obtained the desired result. Unfortunately, many patients have been denied freedom from complaints or even a cure because the rules of repetition are not known or were disregarded.

A reluctant improvement occurs in long-lasting diseases or in patients who were pretreated with many chemical drugs. As a consequence, the body's ability to self-regulate has been impaired, often even blocked, and a condition called **blocked regulation** results. Medications with a regulation-blocking effect are *psychotropic drugs, corticoids, antibiotics*, and *antiallergic drugs*. When taking the patient's history, we must therefore include questions about long-term consumption of medications that can inhibit the efficacy of other therapeutic methods or make them inaccessible for the body.

Repeated cupping tends to remove the blockage.

Please Note

If the body's regulatory capacity is disturbed, it can happen that no treatment is possible because even the therapeutic stimuli of homeopathic remedies or Bach flower remedies are so strong that the pathological symptoms are intensified to their extreme after any therapy (e.g., extremely high fever, unbearable pain, inflammations becoming more acute). Such patients are desperate and have exhausted the last resort. They call off any therapy after a short time, change therapist, and turn to another treatment method. These patients tolerate the first cupping session surprisingly well and hope for even greater therapeutic success with expected treatment sessions. The therapist also often believes in his or her success until the symptoms recur with increasing intensity after cupping treatments have been repeated in intervals that were too short.

Due to the chronicity and the unforeseeable reactions of the organism, the next cupping session should only be performed after 4–6 weeks in such cases. Even if therapists are often asked to relieve a patient's complaints quickly, they have to remember not to schedule the next cupping session too early, to prevent an overly strong reaction by the diseased organism.

Fortunately, cupping is a method that produces therapeutic stimuli for the disturbed regulatory system and relieves the patient's suffering even after the first application.

Persistence, Intensity, and Localization of Complaints After Cupping

> **Note**
>
> The **persistence** of pre-existing complaints after cupping or even the **appearance of additional complaints** at other locations are **diagnostic indications**, just like the **remission** of complaints at the treatment site or the **appearance of new complaints** at a different place.

In these cases, we always have to consider the possibility that a **remote disturbance** (also, focal disturbance) could be present at the location of the new complaints.

An example from my clinical practice can illustrate this in more detail.

A 50-year-old patient had suffered from severe shoulder and neck pain for three years. Treatment with cups placed on the painful locations brought little improvement. By contrast, she began experiencing intestinal problems. I continued treatment with cupping, but now at the intestinal reflex zones, in conjunction with prescribing homeopathic remedies. Through this treatment, I obtained cure of all complaints.

Thus, we can see that not every shoulder pain indicates rheumatism or arthritis and that not all heart trouble is an indication for disease in this organ. Shoulder pain can originate in disease of the intestines, heart, or lungs, for example, or even in changes in the cervical spinal column, and heart trouble can also be triggered by a diseased thyroid gland.

> **Note**
>
> Intensification of pre-existing complaints, especially of pain, is also a diagnostic sign.

We can observe this type of effect in patients with **vasodilatory tendencies**. In such patients, application of warmth causes the condition to worsen, but application of cold brings relief.

> **Memorize** **M!**
>
> In such cases, cupping has no benefit!

The following is an additional diagnostic indication:

> **Note**
>
> Chills or shivering that appear after cupping but recede after a short bedrest suggest a chronic (often protracted) focal disturbance.

Finally, cupping allows us to differentiate between **neurasthenic syndrome** and *vegetative dystonia*. In patients with **neurasthenic syndrome**, an initial cupping treatment tends to result in an obvious improvement, if not disappearance, of existing complaints, but **only for a short time**. In such cases, repeated treatments do not bring further improvement of the condition. Patients even complain of drastic aggravation.

Neither do we see any new symptoms that could potentially indicate a focal disturbance. Treatments with other naturopathic methods follow the same pattern. In patients with neurasthenic syndrome, we often come across a nervous breakdown in their previous medical history.

Memorize	M!
For this disease, cupping is ineffective.	

In patients with **vegetative dystonia**, on the other hand, the initial treatment will only bring unsatisfactory improvement of the stated complaints for the patient. No additional symptoms appear either, if it is indeed a case of clear functional disregulation of the vegetative nervous system without an organic primary disease.

Patients with **vegetative dystonia** respond well, even if only reluctantly, to repeated cupping treatments. The cups should be placed on the sites of the stated complaints as well as on top of the spinal column.

Supplemental therapies also show excellent results.

6.1.5 Segmental Diagnosis (Head's Zones)

Diagnostic keys are not limited to the manifestations described above but also include extravasates formed in Head's zones.

The following illustration (▶ Fig. 6.1) shows in which segment we are likely to see reactions are transferred from the associated internal organs to the trunk muscles and skin.

Note
Segmental diagnosis can always only suggest *at which location* a disturbance is present. It is, however, unable to indicate the name or cause of the disease.

6.2 Clinical Application

6.2.1 Materials and Basic Equipment

Suction cups, also called cupping jars, are round glass cups of varying sizes with a slightly narrower neck. Different models of suction cups exist (▶ Fig. 6.2).

I personally follow the old method of creating a vacuum in the cups by heating and thereby thinning the air with a flame. In my opinion, this old way of creating a vacuum by applying heat and then letting the air cool off is much more effective than the cupping vessels available today, in which a vacuum can be created by means of a rubber ball or plunger pump. Furthermore, the warm air in the cup causes an additional stimulus on the skin.

Anybody who wants to look into the art of cupping should have suction cups of varying sizes in their clinic.

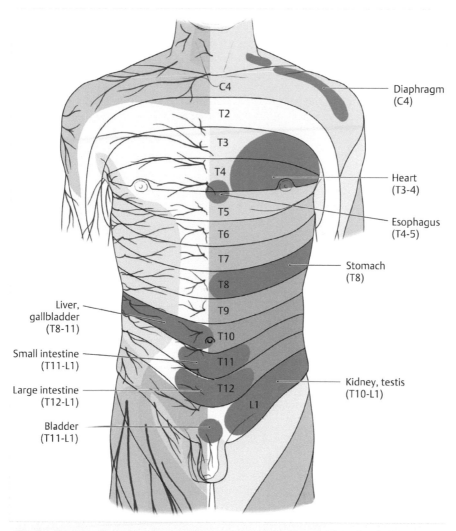

Fig. 6.1 Orienting illustration of segmental association of the internal organs (Head's zones). (Schünke M, Schulte E, Schumacher U. THIEME Atlas of Anatomy. Head, Neck, and Neuroanatomy. Illustrations by M. Voll and K. Wesker. 3rd ed. Stuttgart: Thieme; 2020)

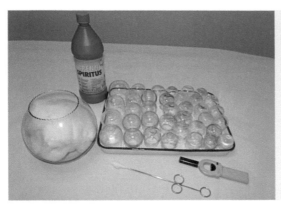

Fig. 6.2 Suction cups and accessories.

For cupping, you need:
• Alcohol.
• A cotton ball that is held, for example, with a surgical clamp.
• A container with water.
• An alcohol burner.

6.2.2 Cupping Technique

Cupping is easy to perform. There are several techniques for placing the suction cups. The following cupping technique by means of a flame of fire is simple and proven.

At the beginning of cupping, dip the cotton ball into the bottle of alcohol until it is soaked and then gently squeeze it out at the bottle rim to prevent excess alcohol from falling down in the form of burning drops. Now you light the cotton ball, take a suction cup into your hand, and insert the burning cotton ball as quickly as possible and as close to the treatment site as possible into the cup and back out again (▶ Fig. 6.3).

You should not heat the cup itself, but only the air inside.

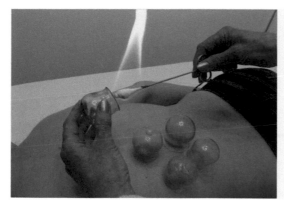

Fig. 6.3 Heating the air inside a suction cup.

When treating large areas of skin with cupping, the patient should lie down during treatment. Nevertheless, there are also cupping sites for which the patient must be treated sitting upright (e.g., the shoulder joint).

Body hair must be shaved off at the cupping sites. In addition, you should pay attention to the patient's and your own hair to prevent potential damage by the fire.

6.3 Individualized and Patient-Centered Application

6.3.1 Cupping Therapy on Children

The technique for cupping on children is the same as described above. It is, however, best to use *small suction cups.*

There is no minimum age for cupping therapy that a child should have reached to avoid potential side-effects and harm, as we are used to for chemical drugs or therapies in conventional Western medicine. I have, for example, on several occasions in my own clinic treated newborn babies only a few days old with excellent results by applying two cups on the back to cure a serious cold and simultaneously prevent pneumonia.

With increasing age of the child, you can also use more cups and place them at different locations. What is different, though, is the way in which you prepare the child **before** the cupping session. As we all know, children tend to be afraid of fire and unknown procedures that could cause them pain. This also applies to the first cupping treatment.

It is a serious mistake to try to force treatment onto a child since it is rather easy to get a child to agree to a treatment without any coercion. We simply have to show and explain that cupping does not hurt but that you only feel how the skin is getting pulled into the suction cup.

It is also appropriate to show the child how the cups are applied by performing this first on your own body at the thigh. Afterwards, you can place the cup on the same location at the child's body. This experience convinces the child that cupping does not hurt and that the cup is not hot even though we have worked with fire.

When you apply cups to the chest, you should ask children to close their eyes so that they will not see the fire near their body. Incidentally, this also applies to adults.

After preparing children in this way, I have never had any problems.

6.3.2 Cupping Therapy on Elderly and Bedridden Patients

Elderly Patients

Aging is a natural and irreversible biological process that starts at birth. In every age, there are constructive and deconstructive processes of individual cells. After the age of 50, however, deconstructive processes become dominant.

Degenerative processes in the organism manifest in deteriorating bodily functions:
- Reduced adaptability of the body, for example to cold or heat.
- Weakened resistance to infectious diseases.
- Decreased secretion of digestive fluids.

The metabolism slows down, and toxins build up in the bodily fluids and tissue, which already have a slower metabolism due to insufficient circulation. This accumulation of toxins is further promoted by insufficient detoxification by the liver and insufficient elimination by the kidneys.

Age-related changes can at any time also cause changes or failure of an organ with corresponding diseases.

While aging is not a disease, the changed self-regulation of the body requires that any therapist adjusts treatment methods correspondingly. They must not cause additional strain on the aging organism. For this reason, the use of chemical drugs should be reduced to a minimum.

Cupping, on the other hand, can be deployed in a supplemental fashion, in which case it is able to substantially reduce the consumption of chemical drugs. Improved circulation accelerates the metabolism and detoxification, as a result of which complaints are relieved more quickly.

Memorize **M!**

The cupping procedure is identical to that described in the section on "Cupping Technique" above. It is important to note that aging manifests in thinner and drier skin and in reduced muscle tissue. You should therefore make it a habit to rub the skin with oil (e.g., massage oil, castor oil) before a cupping treatment.

> **Note**
>
> Nevertheless, **treatment intervals** differ from those for young patients because of declining regulatory and regenerative processes and delayed speed of nerve conduction.

The following treatment course has therefore proven effective in the treatment of older patients:

> **Memorize**   **M!**
>
> - Initially, three treatments per week are required.
> - Experience shows that patients already feel an effect after the first treatment. As a consequence, confidence in the therapy is strengthened and this motivates them to continue.
> - Obvious improvement generally occurs after about six treatment sessions.
> - Until complaints have completely disappeared, one treatment per week is necessary.
> - Repeated treatments are essential to sustain the achieved results.

In the course of time, patients will first ask for cupping treatments also for other complaints.

> **Note**
>
> Combination with other types of therapies is always appropriate.

Bedridden Patients

Nursing patients in need of care must not be limited to the necessary daily tasks or to human affection and goodwill, but must also include preventative strengthening of the immune defense system. Because of impaired circulation, a bedridden patient tends to suffer not only from bedsores but also from pain in the back and chest regions, as well as from dangerous cases of *pneumonia,* especially after surgery and in older patients.

In my opinion, cupping is an outstanding tool for at least reducing the above-mentioned additional problems in cases of week-long bedrest. This is especially true because the circulation not only of the skin, but also of the lung and pleura can be affected greatly by cupping. In addition, one or several cupping treatments after surgery can make the use of antibiotics unnecessary and also shorten the period of recovery.

The application of the cups in bedridden patients is identical to the standard procedures. The only difference lies in the way in which you handle the bedridden patient.

In cases of irreversible disturbances, cupping does not provide a cure, but it improves the patient's quality of life.

6.3.3 Exceptional Cases During Cupping and the Correct Response

To avoid panicking that cupping could have done harm or caused one of the indications listed below as a result of incorrect application, we must be aware of the following:

Small blisters filled with lymph can form at the cupping site. I have observed this most commonly in patients with very sensitive skin.

If they have burst on their own, treat the spots carefully with a disinfectant. They generally disappear within a day.

In very thin patients, more or less **severe pain** can arise immediately after cupping at the treatment sites, or **clotted, knot-like spots** can form in the subcutaneous tissue. These manifestations can be remedied with oil (e.g., massage oil, castor oil), even after cupping.

In such cases, this is not a harmful effect of cupping itself, but a perfectly normal reaction, caused by the lack of storage fat.

It is possible that the cups **fail to suck** at all or **continue to fall off** in locations where the muscles are very tense (e.g., in the neck) or where a large amount of lymph fluid has accumulated in the soft parts of the body or the interstitial tissue. Please, do not lose your patience, but continue to try placing the cups on the same spot! If they have fallen off three times at a place with tensed muscles, apply cupping massage to relax the muscles.

A few hints, also for standard cases, to complete this list:

- In **rheumatic disorders** or **neural inflammations**, heat has an additional therapeutic effect. In such cases, you can rub the skin before cupping with a warming ointment, provided that the patient tolerates this.
- **After cupping**, the patient does not need to remain in bed if the condition itself does not require this (as for example, in common cold or pneumonia).

- **Briefly massaging** the **cupping sites** after cupping causes even faster and stronger results. This should, however, not be done on weakened patients.
- Cupping may also **be performed daily** (e.g., drying up of lymph fluid accumulations in the interstitial spaces), but never in a place where a hematoma is still visible.
- **Hematomas that persist for too long** (ca. 1 week) may be treated with an ointment that promotes reabsorption.

6.4 The Technique of Cupping Massage

Massage as such has been used as a form of therapy for thousands of years. In our times, it has acquired strict anatomical foundations and as a result, we obtain excellent results with specifically directed massage.

An alternative form of massage is one that utilizes a **suction cup**. This is a specialized technique that functions, just like cupping itself, as segmental and regulation therapy. It also produces hyperemia and extravasates.

> **Note**
>
> This type of treatment has a deeper effect than traditional hand massage.

Cupping massage has the effect of increasing circulation throughout the treatment site, promoting metabolism, and therefore the nourishment of tissue there. In addition, cupping massage removes accumulated flakes of epidermis and thereby increases its permeability and skin respiration.

The effects of cupping massage on the muscles are more mechanical: by promoting the drainage of blood and lymph, it stimulates the metabolism and has a positive effect on the body as a whole. The body's resistance is strengthened and self-regulation of the disturbed bodily functions is initiated.

Almost all disorders and muscular changes are approachable with cupping massage.

> **Note**
>
> Its primary application, however, is in the realm of localized muscle tension. It is one of the best procedures for relaxing and loosening.

Nevertheless, cupping massage not only influences the directly treatable tissue (skin, muscles), but also, as cupping itself via the reflex pathways the internal organs.

The **indications for cupping massage** are basically identical to those of cupping. It is particularly suited for the following conditions:

- Muscle disorders.
- Impaired circulation.
- Headache/migraine.
- Rheumatic and arthritic joint disorders.
- Disorders of the spinal column.
- Acne.
- Neuralgic pains.

- Bronchial asthma (good results by cupping massage in combination with standard cupping therapy).

6.4.1 Cupping Technique

For **sliding the cup,** apply **massage oil** or **ointment** to the surface of the skin at the treatment site. Then place the suction cup on the skin as in dry cupping and push and pull it on the body surface, possibly also moving it in circles.

When the skin at the treatment site has turned **reddish or bluish,** finish the massage. Hereby, extravasates can form on the whole treated area. The **massage lasts approximately 3 minutes.**

Sometimes the **suction cup falls off** repeatedly during the massage. In spite of this, you can continue with the massage, employing the cup with light pressure as in standard treatments.

It is also possible that a massage, even if performed correctly, causes only slight or **no hyperemia (redness) at all** or instead causes a **bluish coloration of the skin.** In this case, **under no circumstances extend the duration of the massage.** This absence of a visible treatment effect generally occurs at areas of the body with poor circulation. The tissue is still loosened at these places, even if we do not see any redness, and the patient experiences the cupping massage as heating.

It is a common occurrence that **cupping massage** causes pain during the massage, similar to that from a strong connective tissue massage.

Also after the massage, pain that resembles muscle stiffness after exertion can occur. If it does not disappear quickly on its own but causes discomfort, it can be remedied quite easily with warm showers or hot compresses.

6.4.2 Diagnostic Hint

The place that is most tender during a cupping massage points to the *locus of the disease.*

If we see additional complaints at a completely different location after the massage, these are thus an indication of a *remote disturbance.*

6.5 Indications for Dry Cupping

The therapeutic applications of cupping are quite extensive because it is not rooted in the pharmacological effect of a few medications but affects the organism as a whole in the sense of stimulus therapy. For individual disorders, see Part 3.

6.6 Contraindications for Dry Cupping

There are only few cases where dry cupping is contraindicated:
- In pregnant women **up to the fourth month of pregnancy**, dry cupping should not be performed (risk of miscarriage!).
- Limited therapy in **tuberculosis** and all kinds of **tumors** is advisable. Here, we must not, of course, place any cups on those sections of the skin that are located above the tumors or organs affected by tuberculosis. Nevertheless, dry cupping on other parts of the body is allowed.

7 Wet Cupping

7.1 Technique and Clinical Advice

Like bloodletting, wet cupping is a type of *blood-extracting therapy*.

It works not only by extracting blood, but also by dissipating and regulating. The regulating effect is caused by two factors. First, the loss of blood serves as a stimulus to the bone marrow and initiates the formation of new erythrocytes as well as an increase in leukocytes. Second, the withdrawal of blood changes the quality of the blood, for example, by reducing viscosity and thereby improving its properties of flow, which has a positive effect on the tissue environment and corresponding biochemical processes.

The result is a general stimulation of the entire organism.

Three methods exist for performing bloody cupping.

7.1.1 Method A

In the first option, the location on the skin where blood is to be extracted is cleaned with a disinfectant and the scarificator (▶ Fig. 7.1) is positioned firmly. The blades simultaneously produce several small incisions, 1 cm long and 4 mm deep. The suction cup is placed on top of these as in dry cupping, to suck the blood out of the scratch wounds.

7.1.2 Method B

In the second version of wet cupping, locations that have just been treated with dry cupping are cleaned with a disinfectant and the cupping site is then scratched with the **scarificator**. After this, the suction cups are positioned on the **same locations**.

Allow the cups to suck for **10–15 minutes**.

A suction cup sucks **ca. 20 mL of blood**. Depending on how much blood you want to extract, conclude the extraction of blood after the first cupping session or place the cups back again on the same locations.

The amount of blood to be extracted depends for the most part on the patient's pathologic condition, age, constitution, and state of health. Normally, you extract ca. **50–300 mL** of blood, that is, you use **2–15 medium-sized suction cups**.

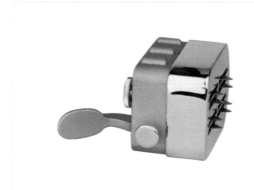

Fig. 7.1 Scarificator.

After cupping is finished, you swab the skin again with a **disinfectant** and dress it with **ointment and a bandage**. The patient should **rest for up to 20 minutes** afterwards.

If required, wet cupping can be repeated in **intervals of 4–8 weeks**.

Note

In wet cupping, disinfection, sterilization, and the use of disposable gloves must be a matter of course.

Memorize   **M!**

For wet cupping, note the following: Do not perform blood cupping above the vertebrae, on the front of the thorax, or in the vicinity of large veins.

In standard cases, blood cupping is performed on sitting patients. Nevertheless, in very sensitive patients you can **also perform cupping lying down**, but this complicates the removal of the blood-filled cups.

To determine whether a certain location on the skin may be treated with wet cupping, carry out a **massage test**. Lubricate the area well with oil and massage with a suction cup. If a few movements produce **redness** or **extravasates**, this indicates that wet cupping may be performed here.

In most cases, a wet cupping session is followed by a general feeling of weakness and a tendency to sweating. The relieving effect of cupping soon takes over in the form of sleepiness and heightened well-being.

7.1.3 Method C—Alternative to the Scarificator

Since ancient times, blood cupping has been performed by using a scarificator, which makes several cuts at once on the indicated skin area. Because this process creates small scars on the scarification site, bloody cupping is rarely used today. As a result, demand for the manufacturing of scarificators has also dropped. Nevertheless, bloody cupping continues to be a procedure with great benefits for the disorders listed in the following section. To avoid scarring the skin, a thin cannula or blood lancet can be used to stab the skin repeatedly and quickly, after which a cup is applied. Soon, you can observe how the blood is pulled up into the glass. The amount of blood drawn in this way is, however, less than when a scarificator is used. To increase the amount of blood, you should remove the cupping glass after a short time and apply a new cup, to increase the suctioning effect. You can count on a blood loss of 30–60 mL.

7.2 Indications for Wet Cupping

In contrast to applications in earlier times, when wet cupping was used excessively, we now have exact indications, such as acute cases of pulmonary congestion as a result of cardiac insufficiency. The extraction of blood reduces the amount of blood in the patient and thereby relieves the strain on the heart muscle. In addition, the life-threatening blood congestion inside the lung can be critically improved.

Wet cupping is also an option in:
- Apoplexy.
- Bronchial asthma, chronic, if it is not purely allergic.
- High blood pressure.
- States of severe fever (pneumonia, influenza).
- Gastritis.
- Headache.
- Polyemia (polycythcmia) etc.

Given that the indication has been determined with precision, the results of cupping treatment appear very quickly. Combinations with other naturopathic methods are always possible.

For individual disorders, see Part 3.

7.3 Complications and Contraindications for Wet Cupping

Wet cupping is **contraindicated** in:
- Tuberculosis of the lung.
- Neoplasms.
- Hypotonia.
- Hemophilia.
- Anemic conditions.
- Menstruation.
- Deficiency of fluids, for example, in severe diarrhea.
- Children, adolescents, the elderly, very sensitive persons with tendency to fainting.
- Arrhythmia.
- Coronary insufficiency with anginal complaints.

Memorize	M!
Great care is necessary in patients with a tendency to stronger bleeding than normal. It is even better in such cases to refrain from wet cupping.	

Due to the performed scarification of the skin, *mild* pain is possible and scars can form. We should not forget that the formation of scars, even if they are only small, is basically not a harmless side-effect for the organism. According to the principles of Huneke therapy, scars can have such a strong effect of permanent stimulation on the neurovegetative system that it is disturbed.

Before reaching for the scarificator, the therapist should consider these points and educate the patient accordingly.

Part 3

Cupping Therapy of Indicated Disorders and Complaints

8 Comments on the Organization and Use of this Part

Given precise determination of indications, you will accomplish successful therapy, even in cases that have been previously treated in clinic without success.

G. Bachmann

Cupping offers effective assistance in the treatment of both minor and major complaints in almost any naturopathic clinic. Nevertheless, before reaching for the cups, we must learn the technique of cupping and familiarize ourselves with its indications and contraindications. In addition, correct location is important in cupping and is one of the crucial factors for its efficacy.

Any treatment method, even a very simple one, may lead to failure or accidents if the basic rules are not known. For example, herbal teas consumed *in excess,* or *incorrectly applied* cold or warm compresses can do more harm than good.

Cupping will often suffice on its own to improve or even eliminate complaints. In other cases that may seem identical on the surface, you must bring in a different therapeutic method as primary, supplemental, or adjunctive therapy.

> **Note**
>
> Cupping is an ideal method for combining with other therapeutic processes.

In many cases, as for example in any acute disease caused by **pathogens**, you have to deploy **antibiotics** as the remedy for fighting the pathogens. In this case, cupping plays a key supportive role as a complementary therapy. It facilitates a quicker and stronger effect of the antibiotics, as a result of which the course of the disease is shortened and the amount of chemical drugs can be reduced.

In this chapter, I list all disorders that can be treated with cupping therapy, also naming the associated cupping sites, and illustrating them with photographs. Herein, the number of suction cups represents an approximate mean that can be increased or decreased in accordance with individual needs.

> **Memorize** **M!**
>
> Depending on cupping site and body size, dry cupping requires 2–35 medium-sized cups, while wet cupping requires 2–15, depending on the amount of blood to be extracted.

It is only with reservations that suggestions for therapy can be offered, since a flexible approach that takes the stage of the disease and the patient's state of health into consideration is absolutely necessary.

> **Note**
>
> The *cupping intervals* indicated for individual disorders only apply to *dry cupping.*
> For *wet cupping,* the standard *interval between cupping sessions is 4 to 8 weeks.*

The supplemental therapies indicated for individual disorders have proven effective as a *complement* to cupping.

The naturopathic methods recommended for alternating application should be regarded as an aid in selecting possible therapies. Decisions on the type and duration of treatment are always up to the therapist.

Every beginning is difficult, but the effort is worth it. Do not get discouraged by initial difficulties.

9 Disorders of the Head

9.1 Headache

Headache is undoubtedly the most common pain disorder that the therapist encounters in CAM practice. The causes of headache are manifold and occur not only in disturbances in the head region, but also as a result or symptom of an internal disease, injury, high blood pressure, allergy, menstruation, or as an early symptom of serious conditions.

The most common causes of headache include:

- States of internal tension. Depression, fear, accumulated aggression, and exhaustion can all tense the muscles of the neck, which can cause headache. Patients, however, also tend to complain of other symptoms such as sleep disorders.
- Excessive muscle tension in the shoulder and neck muscles, in connection with poor circulation. We see this commonly in patients who strain their shoulder or neck muscles unilaterally or spend time in drafty rooms.
- Disorders of the spinal column.

Because headaches are always a symptom and not a disease, we must first clarify their cause, for example, high blood pressure, liver disease, or allergy.

9.1.1 Symptoms

Headache that is caused by muscle tension or disorders of the spinal column:

- Often persistent headache.
- Location is mostly in the areas of the neck/back of the head, radiating to the forehead.
- Sensation of cold.

Caution! ⚠
Resistant to pain-killers. Relief of pain by warmth, massage.

9.1.2 Suggested Therapy

In standard cases, a single cupping session (▶ Fig. 9.1) will be sufficient. If necessary, **one treatment daily for up to 4 days.**

Note
In patients with severe pain, supplemental therapy (neural therapy) is indicated. In headaches where the source is found in hypertonia or hyperemia, wet cupping is recommended: paravertebral in segments **C3–C5**.

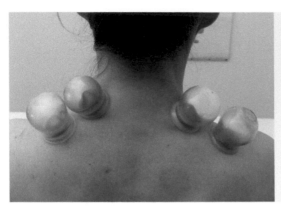

Fig. 9.1 Dry cupping in the neck and shoulder region in segments C4–C6, especially in points that are sensitive to pressure. Do not place the cups on top of the cervical spine.

9.2 Migraine

Migraine is a particular type of headache. You should, however, only make the diagnosis of migraine when you are dealing with the strictly outlined clinical picture for this disease.

Migraine presents a clearly definable clinical picture whose typical symptoms allow a diagnosis with great certainty. Possible triggers are:

- The psyche.
- Frequently at the onset of menstruation.
- Certain foods.
- The effects of weather.
- Lack of sleep.

9.2.1 Symptoms

There is usually a sudden onset of an attack with half- or double-sided headache, pulsing, severe, aggravated by light and noise, located mostly in the temples or forehead-orbital region, and often accompanied by flickering lights before the eyes, nausea, and vomiting.

9.2.2 Suggested Therapy

In migraine attacks with vasoconstriction of the vessels, cupping (▶ Fig. 9.2) or cupping massage is the "method of choice" (pain relief through warmth).

In the **vasodilatory stage**, on the other hand, cupping rarely improves the condition (pain relief through cold). In such cases, cupping is of purely diagnostic significance, and you have to employ other therapies, such as **neural therapy**.

Memorize	M!
In migraine, treatment must be initiated early.	

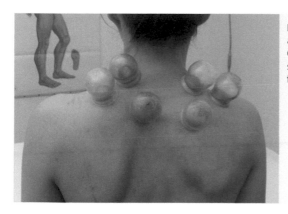

Fig. 9.2 Dry cupping in the neck and shoulder region in segments C3–C6, especially on points that are sensitive to pressure. Do not perform cupping on the cervical spine.

First to third day, one treatment daily. From the fifth day on, treatments should occur **every 5 or 7 days**. Afterwards, intervals between treatments can be increased depending on the results to **14 days at first**, and later to **4 weeks**. Continue treatment long enough to reach the goal.

> **Note**
>
> In migraines with vasodilatory manifestations: wet cupping in segments C3-T4.

9.2.3 Supplemental Therapy

- Depending on the case: **Psychotherapy.**
- **Phytotherapy**. Plant-based psychotropic drugs, for example, St. John's wort.
- **Autogenic training.**
- **Homeopathy**. This disease is very diverse in terms of triggers and manifestations, and also closely related to the disposition and condition of the patient. Hence migraine requires a very precise response and the choice of a far-reaching remedy. In cases where the treatment of migraine is ineffective, you have either chosen the wrong remedy or the wrong diagnosis.
- **Neural therapy**. In patients with severe pain, quaddle therapy with local anesthetics is indicated as supplemental therapy.

9.2.4 Alternating Therapy

- **Neural therapy**. Migraine in the *vasodilatory stage* and in severe headache.
- **Acupuncture**. Migraine in *severe cases,* intermittent treatment, acute treatment.
- **Electroacupuncture**. Can be helpful for **vasomotoric pain**.

9.3 Middle Ear Inflammation (Otitis Media)

The inner ear and the auditory nerve can be affected by certain disorders that have started anywhere in the body. The middle ear, however, is most susceptible to inflammation, which tends to be caused by an infection ascending from the nasopharyngeal region.

Inflammations of the middle ear occur particularly often in infants and toddlers due to special characteristics of their anatomy. The prevention of otitis media depends on how fast you bring infections in the nose and throat into remission.

9.3.1 Symptoms

- Suddenly occurring stabbing pain in the ear.
- Occasional tinnitus, fever.
- Temporarily also loss of hearing.
- Degraded general condition.
- Headache.

9.3.2 Suggested Therapy

Cupping is most effective in accordance with the following formula:
- **Acute stage**. One treatment per day for 2 days.
- **Chronic stage**. Here, treatments occur only every 3 or 5 days. Continue these long enough to ensure that the goal is reached.

> **Note**
>
> See ▶ Fig. 9.2: Dry cupping in the neck and shoulder region in segments **C3–C6**.

9.4 Tinnitus

The ear is an organ in which arteries terminate. As such, it reacts with particular sensitivity to poor circulation. Three conditions related to the blood supply of the inner ear are **noises in the ear, defective hearing**, and **dizziness**.

If the complaints alternate and are characterized by a recurrent, acute nature, we must consider poor circulation and its effects (e.g., in cervical syndrome irritation of the sympathetic fibers with tissue spasms).

Further possible causes include:
- Excessive doses of chemical drugs, such as acetylsalicylic acid (aspirin), diuretics, cytostatics, and many others.
- Degenerative disorders of the central nervous system and inner ear.
- Trauma, for example, noise trauma.
- Metabolic diseases, for example, diabetes mellitus, hypothyroidism, avitaminosis, kidney disease.

9.4.1 Symptoms

Ringing, humming, rustling, whistling, or other noises in the head are generally related to the inner ear.

9.4.2 Suggested Therapy

Treatment only after the cause is determined. In tinnitus, any therapy promises success that is able to remedy the nerve irritation and poor circulation.

> **Note**
>
> The efficacy of cupping in conditions with poor circulation is well known.

Treatment is recommended according to the following formula:

Initially, **two to three treatments per week**, approximately 15 treatments in total. Following this, **one treatment per week** to sustain the result.

> **Note**
>
> See ▶ Fig. 9.2: Dry cupping in the neck and shoulder region in segments **C3–C6**. Wet cupping in plethoric patients in segments C3 and C6.

9.4.3 Supplemental Therapy

Depending on the case, if necessary **antibiotic therapy.**

> **Caution!**
>
> Treatment with antibiotics often conceals the symptoms of otitis.

- **Homeopathy**: Ear infections are a common disorder with sudden onset in sensitive children. Decisive in homeopathy are the causes, circumstances, and perceptions. Beginning otitis, however, responds well to organotropic therapy.
- **Neural therapy**: Treatment attempt—in severe pain, possibly additionally with quaddle therapy with local anesthetics. Local anesthetics, warmed up to body temperature, as drops.
- **Phytotherapy**: In poor circulation, preparations of special extracts.

9.4.4 Alternating Therapy

- **Chiropractic**: In appropriate cases.
- **Neural therapy**: Quaddle therapy with local anesthetics into cutanovisceral reflex paths, in the area of the cervical segments C2-C3 on both sides of the spinous processes and behind the earlobe on places sensitive to pressure.
- **Baunscheidt therapy**: In the neck and shoulder region.
- **Acupuncture**: Causal therapy depending on cause.

9.5 Sinus Infection (Sinusitis)

An acute or chronic inflammation of the sinuses can affect a single sinus, but can also spread from one sinus to another, ultimately affecting all sinuses. Possible complications are inflammations of the middle ear or lymph nodes, bronchitis, and asthma.

9.5.1 Symptoms

Acute Sinusitis

Acute sinusitis can arise suddenly or gradually as an independent infection or in the course of other infections of the upper respiratory tracts. Additionally, an abscess in the root of a tooth can act as cause of an acute inflammation in the sinuses.

Symptoms are:
- Headache, aggravated by bending down.
- Sensitivity to tapping and pressure above the affected sinuses.
- Fever.
- Nasal congestion.
- Occasionally dizziness and sensitivity to light.

Chronic Sinusitis

The chronic form of sinusitis generally develops from an acute sinusitis that has not been cured. Diseased teeth as well as climatic conditions also promote a latent chronic development of sinusitis.

In the chronic form, complaints are not that severe. Headache occurs primarily in the morning and during the day. Mucous or purulent discharge from the nose; often, the throat is also involved. Breathing through the nose is impeded.

By locating the already existing headache, we can determine which sinus is inflamed or affected the most:
- Pain in the forehead, above and behind the eyes, which occurs in the morning, points to frontal sinusitis.
- Pain in the upper teeth and cheeks, which becomes more severe mostly in the afternoon, is often triggered by a maxillary sinusitis.
- Sphenoid and ethmoid sinusitis generally cause radiating pain in the back of the head, in the vertex area, and in the neck.

9.5.2 Suggested Therapy

In my opinion, cupping is the most effective treatment method for sinusitis. In frontal sinusitis (▶ Fig. 9.3), the application of cupping has an obvious drastic effect, resulting in the disappearance of pain after a single treatment, without chemical drugs, in a short time. Effects are not as immediate in inflammations of the other sinuses, but you will also be successful in causes that have already undergone lengthy previous treatment.

In sphenoid and ethmoid sinusitis, dry cupping in the neck and shoulder area has proven effective (see ▶ Fig. 9.2). This treatment can be repeated after potentially recurring pain.

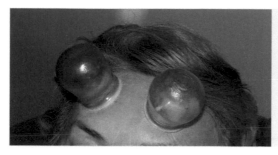

Fig. 9.3 Dry cupping on the forehead in frontal sinusitis. In maxillary sinusitis, dry cupping on the cheeks and below the lower jaw. For this purpose, place two medium-sized cups on the forehead and up to three cups on the affected location. Duration of cupping up to 10 minutes.

Memorize **M!**

When cupping is performed on the face, make sure that no blisters form. Because the skin of the face is considerably thinner than the skin on other parts of the body, you should rub oil into the skin before any cupping session, to prevent blistering. Hematomas, which are unavoidable in most cases of treating inflammation, can be concealed with a blemish stick if the patient is unable to remain at home for a few days.

9.5.3 Supplemental Therapy

Depending on the case:
- If necessary, **antibiotics**.
- If maxillary sinusitis is caused by diseased teeth, treatment success depends first on the **treatment of the teeth.**
- **Regulation therapy**. Can be effective in chronic forms of sinusitis because this often means that the organism's resistance to infections is weakened.
- **Steam baths**. With an infusion of chamomile, yarrow flowers, and thyme.
- **Homeopathy**. Experience shows that the choice of remedy depends on the location, type, and time of onset of the pain, as well as on the type of secretion.

10 Respiratory Tract

10.1 Bronchial Asthma

Bronchial asthma has different causes. It can arise following influenza or pneumonia or in chronic disease of the throat and nose. In addition to chronic catarrhs of the airways, hypersensitivity (allergic reaction) is a key factor in asthma. Psychological or nervous causes (psychological tension or stress, fear, fright, etc.) are also significant. Climate and weather conditions, lastly, have a triggering and boosting effect.

Regardless of the mechanism by which it formed, episodes manifest in shortness of breath, caused by cramp-like bronchial spasms with simultaneous swelling of the bronchial mucous membrane and increased discharge of mucus.

10.1.1 Symptoms

- Episodic, often unexpectedly arising shortness of breath, often with warning signs, such as tickling in the nose, irritation in the larynx.
- It is characteristic that it is not so much inhalations, but mostly exhalations that are severely impeded. In so-called *nervous asthma,* on the other hand, deep inhalations are impeded.
- A typical sign is shortness of breath with yawning and symptom-free intervals.
- Coughing and mucous sputum are concomitant symptoms.

If you have ever observed or even personally experienced the agony of an asthmatic struggling for breath, you will be unable to pass up a request for treatment in cases of bronchial asthma. Continuous treatment of bronchial asthma with *cortisone,* however, invariably causes serious side effects. By contrast, treatment must employ all forms of therapy that are suitable for having a curative effect on bronchial asthma without causing harm.

10.1.2 Suggested Therapy

In acute cases, you can substantially alleviate or even end an asthma attack by cupping (▶ Fig. 10.1 and ▶ Fig. 10.2). Repeated treatments have often succeeded in regulating the entire organism and contributed to recovery.

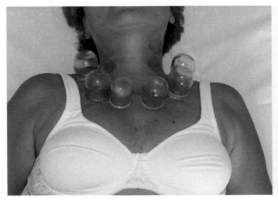

Fig. 10.1 Dry cupping frontally next to the breastbone, also above and below the collar bone.

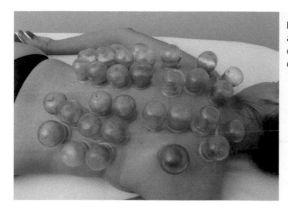

Fig. 10.2 Dry cupping in the neck and shoulder region, on both sides of the thoracic spinal column, and on the lateral sections of the thorax.

The following treatment formula has proven effective. It does, however, require perseverance on the part of the patient:

Initially, intervals should be **5–7 days long** each, for approximately **6 weeks.**

Subsequently, treatment must be continued for at least **1 year in intervals of 2–3 weeks.**

10.1.3 Supplemental Therapy

- **Autourine therapy (AUT).** My experience has taught me that urine, administered orally, is most reliable.
- **Homeopathy.** This disease requires long-term treatment, with the goal of affecting the constitution. Personotropic therapy is based on the discovery that a person's disposition can be affected by individual-specific constitutional remedies.
- **Vitamin and mineral preparations**. Vitamin C, calcium.
- **Oxygen therapy**. Individually adjusted to the specific case and patient's condition.
- **Climatotherapy**. On the North Sea coast, it often results in a regulation of the entire organism and hence a decrease in asthmatic disposition.

10.1.4 Alternating Therapy

- **Neural therapy.** Quaddle therapy with local anesthetic on both sides of the breastbone and above the shoulder as well as on the back along both sides of the thoracic spinal column.
- **Acupuncture**. According to the predominant symptoms at the time.

10.2 Bronchial Catarrh (Bronchitis)

10.2.1 Symptoms

Acute Bronchitis

By acute bronchitis, we mean an inflammation of the mucous membrane in the bronchi, which generally arises subsequent to colds or infections of the upper respiratory tract. The disease can, however, also be caused by inhalation of dust or gases that irritate the mucous membrane.

- Nasal congestion and hoarseness.
- Moderately strong feeling of general malaise, headache.
- Agonizing cough, often dry.
- Slightly elevated temperature.
- When the windpipe is affected, scratching and sensation of soreness behind the breastbone.
- Usually from the third day on ejection of mucous purulent sputum.

Chronic Bronchitis

Chronic bronchitis is an advanced stage of repeatedly occurring acute bronchial catarrh or other diseases as well as of chronic damages that irritate the mucous membranes.
  Symptoms are:

- Cough and expectoration are the first, usually weather-dependent symptoms, with the largest amount of sputum expectorated in the morning.
- Frequently shortness of breath.
- Rarely fever.
- Sensitivity to catching cold.

Because chronic bronchitis initially compromises the patient's general health only slightly, he or she often fails to take it seriously, in spite of the fact that the condition can turn into bronchial asthma.

Because of its positive properties, cupping lends itself also as a supplemental and supportive treatment to methods of conventional Western medicine. It has a stimulating effect on the blood flow, a regulating effect on circulation, and a general regulating effect.

10.2.2 Treatment of Bronchitis

Timely employed cupping in acute bronchitis visibly shortens its course, makes the use of antibiotics unnecessary in most cases, and prevents a potentially threatening pneumonia.

A beginning bronchitis can be cured with a single treatment. In severe cases, cupping treatment must be repeated on the second or third day. If hematomas are still present, position the cups on locations between the hematomas.

In **acute bronchitis**, and especially in fever, bedrest must be observed.

In **chronic bronchitis**, carry out repeated cupping treatments for recovery. In this case, treatment must, of course, be continued for a longer time period, followed by supplemental therapy.

In **chronic** cases, select intervals of initially **5–7 days for 6 weeks** and then continue treatment with sessions spaced **3 weeks apart,** possibly also 6 weeks.

Following this, intervals can be **lengthened**, depending on results, to **once every 4 weeks** (for approximately 1 year).

> **Note**
>
> See ▶ Fig. 10.1: Dry cupping frontally next to the breastbone, also above and below the collar bone.
> See ▶ Fig. 10.2: Dry cupping in the neck and shoulder region, on both sides of the thoracic spinal column, and on the lateral sections of the thorax.
> For wet cupping, see section Bronchial Asthma.

10.2.3 Supplemental Therapy

- If necessary, **antibiotics**.
- **Homeopathy**: The experiences of the past few years have shown that coughs are occurring more and more frequently like an epidemic. As a result, therapists can prescribe the same remedies for many patients, but not for all of them. In homeopathic therapy, we therefore employ remedies according to symptoms that are appropriate for the acute stage of inflammation. For subsequent treatments, remedies are chosen that are indicated for the key characteristics observed in the cough. In chronic cases, the patient's constitutional properties and the course of the disease have to be understood comprehensively to facilitate the proper selection of suitable remedies.
- **Phytotherapy**: In acute and chronic bronchitis, phytopharmaceuticals with anti-irritant properties are used: tea made from mallow, *Plantago lanceolata,* thyme.
- **Gargling solution** of sage.
- **Steam bath inhalations** with essential oils are recommended.

10.3 Influenza and Influenzal Disorders (Influenzal Bronchitis, Influenzal Pneumonia, Bronchopneumonia)

Many common colds are called influenza even though they are not. A true viral influenza is caused by several strains of the influenza virus. The most important ones are *Influenza A* and *Influenza B viruses,* which in many cases trigger epidemics.

New variations of the virus develop from the pathogens. Therefore, effective and long-lasting prophylaxis by vaccination is difficult. A vaccine can only be developed after a new type has emerged.

10.3.1 Symptoms

- Severe pain in the head, limbs, muscles.
- Fever of up to 39°C (102°F).
- Frequently, lumbago-like back pain.
- Feeling exhausted.
- Catarrh of the mucous membranes, followed by tracheitis with retrosternal pain and cough.

Potential complications of a normal flu include:
- Influenzal bronchitis.
- Influenzal pneumonia.
- Bronchopneumonia.
- Pulmonary edema.
- Pleuritis.
- Otitis.
- Sinusitis.
- Circulatory insufficiency.

Influenza is a kind of viral infection in which causative treatment is rarely possible and cupping is therefore particularly significant. Both simple influenzal infections and severe influenzal pneumonia respond well to treatment by cupping. Temperatures normalize quickly. Symptoms like exhaustion, lack of appetite, and bone and muscle pain, which, as we know, seriously impact the person's feeling of overall health, improve almost instantly. Among others, Bachmann has reported his excellent results with cupping therapy in the treatment of influenzal viruses.

In my practice, I have frequently treated mild and severe cases of influenza with cupping. I was able to nip beginning infections in the bud. In serious cases, cupping can almost work miracles, and in cases with suspected influenzal infection, any outbreak at all is prevented. According to my own experience, cupping can also be recommended for any influenzal infections.

We know that therapists, especially in general practice, are often unable to make an exact diagnosis from the start in beginning infections. It is therefore difficult to employ a specific remedy right away. In such cases, we can quite safely commence therapy with cupping in support of the body's own resistance, since it will frequently result in immediate relief or even recovery on its own, without any danger of masking the clinical picture (with fever-reducing medicines).

10.3.2 Suggested Therapy

In beginning general infections like influenzal conditions, we can generally exert a fast, enduring influence on the organism with a single treatment (► Fig. 10.3):

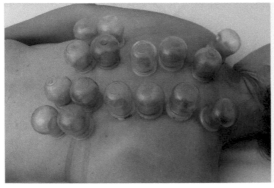

Fig. 10.3 Dry cupping on the entire back. In very thin patients, do not position cups on top of the shoulder blades.

If necessary, the cupping treatment—in front and back—should be **repeated on the second or third day.** In all cases, the patient requires **bedrest for 1–2 days** after cupping.

> **Note**
>
> See ▶ Fig. 10.1: Dry cupping frontally next to the breastbone, also above and below the collar bone.
> In cases with high fever: possibly in addition, wet cupping in segments **T1 -T5.**

10.3.3 Supplemental Therapy

- If necessary, **antibiotics.**
- **Homeopathy.** These disorders are nothing new for the therapist. However, every year the unpredictability of their manifestations is new, that is, the unpredictable effects of triggers like the pathogen type, drenching, hypothermia, drafts, and so on. These disorders require individualized remedy selection in consideration of the overall medical situation.
- **Phytotherapy.** *Expectorant herbal teas* (e.g., thyme, elderflower, linden flower, *Plantago lanceolata,* etc.). Herbs that contain *essential oils* as steam inhalation (e.g., eucalyptus, pine needle, chamomile). *Drugs with tannic acids* as gargling solutions (e.g., oak bark, sage). *Rubs, vitamins (B, C).*
- **In serious cases.** Cardiovascular support, oxygen therapy.

10.3.4 Prophylaxis

- **Homeopathy.** *Influenza nosode* every 14 days in September/October, *Camphora D1* one drop in the morning on a sugar cube from September to April.
- **Phytotherapy.** Plant-based immune stimulants as long-term treatment applied in the early stage. Initiating therapy even in the acute stage is still helpful.
- **Vitamins.**

10.4 Sore Throat (Tonsillitis, Laryngitis, Pharyngitis)

Sore throat arises unexpectedly and acutely as the result of bacterial and viral infections of the sinuses and throat. Sore throat is also an early symptom of a variety of serious diseases such as diphtheria, scarlet fever, and so on, which can bring about serious complications. Correct and timely diagnosis and professional treatment are therefore essential. Sore throat can occur in the following forms.

10.4.1 Symptoms

Tonsillitis

Acute inflammation of the tonsils (angina lacunaris). The disease is most commonly seen in older children and young adults. It is rare in older adults.

- Difficulty swallowing, often with "stinging in the ear."
- Abundant secretion of saliva.
- Fever.
- Headache.
- Exhaustion.

Laryngitis

In most cases, this involves a declining catarrhal inflammation subsequent to a commonplace viral infection. It can also occur after excessive straining of the voice in dry rooms.
   Typical for laryngitis are
- Hoarseness.
- Rough voice.
- Dry cough.
- Tickling or burning in the throat.
- Serious inflammation manifests in pain.

Pharyngitis

This is an inflammation of the mucous membrane of the pharynx, which arises as the result of a general viral infection of the upper respiratory tract.
- Difficulty swallowing.
- Feeling of dryness.
- Itching and burning in the throat.
- In children, fever can concur.

10.4.2 Suggested Therapy

In disorders of the throat (laryngitis, tonsillitis, pharyngitis), cupping treatment is on the lateral sections of the neck (▶ Fig. 10.4). With consistent and properly applied cupping treatments, we can frequently reduce or even discontinue strong medications.

   In the **acute state**, cupping delivers excellent results when applied on time. If it appears necessary, the treatment can be repeated on **the next day**.

   In the **chronic state**, choose **intervals of 7 days** and continue treatment until success is achieved.

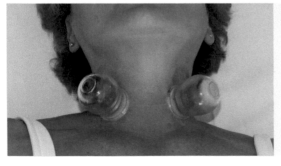

Fig. 10.4 Dry cupping: lateral neck sections.

If the bronchial tubes are involved or in cases of influenza, add cupping therapy in correspondence to existing disorders.

Note
Wet cupping in the neck and shoulder region, in segments C3 and C4.

10.4.3 Supplemental Therapy

- If necessary, **antibiotics**.
- **Homeopathy**. All three disorders generally respond reliably to homeopathic treatment. This is premised, as always, on the proper selection of remedies in accordance with homeopathic principles. In addition to the remedy selection, success with the individual patient also depends on the right potency and dose. The number of possible remedies is relatively small.
- **Phytotherapy**. Phytopharmaceuticals with secretolytic and secretomotoric properties, for example, anise, marshmallow, thyme. Phytopharmaceuticals that contain essential oils, in the form of steam inhalations and gargles.

10.4.4 Alternating Therapy

- **Neural therapy**. Quaddle therapy with local anesthetics in the segment.
- **Acupuncture**. Causal treatment.

10.5 Pneumonia

Pneumonia is an inflammatory disease of the lung tissue, caused by bacteria or viruses. In cases where the inflammation spreads along the bronchial tubes throughout the whole lung, we speak of **bronchopneumonia**. When it only affects a single lobe or section of the lung without transcending its borders, it is called **lobar pneumonia**. Besides influenza, pneumonia is even today still one of the most common diseases.

Pneumonia occurs at any time of the year, but a protracted common cold, another viral disease, any bacterial cold in the nasopharyngeal space all contribute to its formation. Persons with a weakened immune system who are already weakened by previous illness are particularly susceptible. Lack of vitamin C also promotes the creation of this disease.

10.5.1 Symptoms

- Beginning usually with shivering and rapidly rising temperature, up to 40°C (104°F).
- Elevated pulse: up to 120 beats per minute.
- Cutting pain in the chest area, side, or shoulder that becomes unbearable during inhalation.
- Painful cough with sputum that is often reddish-brown in color.
- Breathing is shallow and rapid. The patient suffers from definite feeling of malaise with headache and exhaustion.
- Viral pneumonia usually manifests with constantly changing fever, dry cough, and exhaustion.

10.5.2 Suggested Therapy

Treatment with cupping in beginning or already existing pneumonia clearly shortens its course and reduces the need for antibiotics.

You can also achieve good results with cupping in subacute lung disorders, with the exception of tuberculosis and neoplasms.

In all forms of pneumonia, the patient requires strict bedrest after cupping.

Note

See ▶ Fig. 10.1: Dry cupping frontally next to the breastbone, also above and below the collar bone.

See ▶ Fig. 10.2: Dry cupping in the neck and shoulder region, on both sides of the thoracic spinal column, and on the lateral sections of the thorax.

In high fever and in cases with high blood pressure, the additional application of a few (two to four) wet suction cups in segments **T1-T5** is helpful.

10.5.3 Supplemental Therapy

- In bacterial pneumonia, targeted treatment with **antibiotics**.
- **Homeopathy**: Concurrent homeopathic treatment accelerates recovery. The primary remedy, as well as the appropriate nosode, should be prescribed on the basis of the patient's individual symptoms. Pneumonia treatment is generally quite rewarding.
- **Phytotherapy**: To control the cough, phytopharmaceuticals that strengthen the heart.
- **Vitamins**: Especially Vitamin C.
- **In serious forms**: Cardiovascular assistance and oxygen therapy. Breathing air must be fresh, air out more frequently.

10.5.4 Prophylaxis

Universally valid recommendations for preventing pneumonia do not exist because there is no immunity. One type of prophylaxis is the timely application of cupping therapy in respiratory illnesses and the implementation of a thorough supplemental therapy, in addition to measures for strengthening the immune system.

10.6 Pleurisy

Pleurisy is a common complication in pneumonia, pericardial disorders, chronic bronchial catarrh, and so on, which often remains unnoticed. The disease is caused either by germs traveling in the bloodstream or by inflammations spreading from neighboring organs.

We distinguish between a *dry* form of pleurisy (pleuritis sicca) and a *wet* form (pleuritis exudativa). In *acute* pleurisy, the smooth, moist surfaces of the pleura first become dry and rough. This creates a sound called the pleural friction rub, typical in dry inflammation of the pleura.

Dry pleurisy often devolves into the wet type. In wet pleurisy, 2–3 L of exudate may form in the space between the parietal and visceral pleura, causing the two leaves to stick. This discharge can restrict the lung substantially. As soon as the exudate forms, the sharp pain is displaced by difficulty breathing. Cicatrization, which has arisen during recovery, makes the inflamed surfaces of the pleura more prone to growing together, and a "slab" of pleural scar tissue develops on the affected side. Consequently, the patient becomes short-winded with even minor motions. We often find pockets with leftover exudates in the pleural scar tissue, which are the cause of sudden relapses.

10.6.1 Symptoms

- Begins slowly and then lasts longer—chronic or acute with back and side pain or stitches.
- Irritating cough without phlegm.
- More or less pronounced shortness of breath.
- Fever, chills, and frequent profuse sweating can occur.
- In dry pleurisy, the patient prefers to lie on the healthy side, in wet pleurisy, on the diseased side.

10.6.2 Suggested Therapy

Cupping can so strongly influence circulation in the lung and pleura that the results are noticed immediately.

Pleurisy requires very attentive care, to prevent the formation of pleural scar tissue or other effects. Therefore, cupping treatment should be initiated *as soon as possible* (▶ Fig. 10.5).

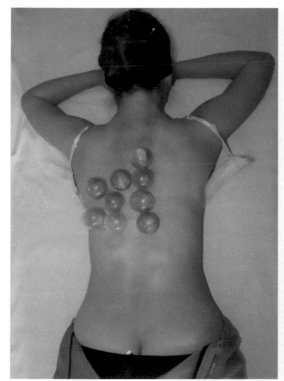

Fig. 10.5 Dry cupping locally on the diseased side and in its vicinity, especially on top of tender points.

In wet pleurisy, daily cupping. As the condition improves, every second or third day up to complete recovery (~2 weeks).

10.6.3 Supplemental Therapy

- **Chemotherapy**, if necessary.
- **Homeopathy**: We can apply several general directives for prescribing a homeopathic remedy, but these can easily be wrong, because for homeopathic therapy, the inflammatory stage is relevant. A few remedies are almost always sufficient for curing ordinary, dry, or exudative pleurisy.
- **Dietetics**: For the prevention of larger effusions, short-term juice or fruit diet in acute stages.

11 Cardiovascular System

11.1 Coronary Heart Disease (Angina Pectoris)

Angina pectoris manifests in episodic painful, oppressive feeling in the area of the heart, retrosternal, or in the upper abdomen. The severe pain of angina pectoris can be caused by a variety of heart disorders, but is most commonly a sign of inadequate blood supply (hypoxia) of the heart muscle, as, for example, in a pathological constriction of the coronary arteries. Constriction of the coronary arteries can have different causes:

- *Arteriosclerotic processes.* Symptoms manifest especially after physical exertion.
- *Nervous disturbances.* A temporary spasmodic constriction of the coronary arteries, especially after states of excitation.
- *Coronary insufficiency in ventricular hypertrophy.* For example, in arterial hypertension or aortic stenosis, certain types of arrhythmia.

11.1.1 Symptoms

- Suddenly occurring "pain of annihilation" in the area of the heart, often radiating to the left shoulder and into the left arm.
- Occasionally also just mild pressure in the area of the heart or epigastrium.
- Fearful feeling, dyspnea, accelerated pulse, arrhythmia.
- During attacks: cool, pale, often sweaty face with fearful expression.
- Occasional provocation of the pain by meals or cold. Sometimes nausea and urinary urgency directly after attacks.
- Duration of attacks: several minutes to half an hour.

11.1.2 Suggested Therapy

During attacks, administering **nitrate preparations** sublingually or as aerosol often offers instant relief. Cupping can obviously not replace nitrate preparations in this case. Nevertheless, nitrate preparations are unable to cause persistent vasodilation, so important in this disease, which is in turn possible with cupping (► Fig. 11.1 and ► Fig. 11.2). Bachmann reports complete cure of angina pectoris with repeated cupping.

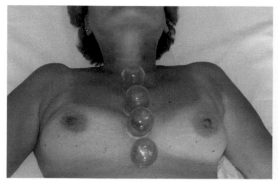

Fig. 11.1 Dry cupping: left parasternal.

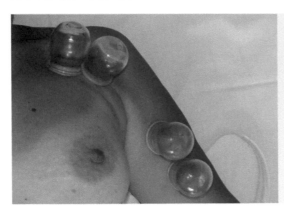

Fig. 11.2 Dry cupping on the inside of the left arm and in the vicinity of the shoulder joint frontally, especially on tender points.

Initially, two to three treatments per week, to a total of 15, that is, the course of treatment lasting 5–7 weeks. **Subsequently, one treatment every 3 weeks.**

Perhaps alternating with cupping massage on the left arm and intercostal area as well as the thorax and shoulder girdle and neck muscles.

11.1.3 Supplemental Therapy

- **Homeopathy.** In this disease, a purely organotropic treatment is possible, in which therapy with constitutional remedies can become necessary. To prevent attacks, we must address the root condition. Depending on the root condition and constitution, a whole series of remedies can be considered.
- **Phytotherapy.** Preparations of special extracts.
- **Autogenic training.** General relaxation, stress reduction.

11.2 Low Blood Pressure (Hypotension)

Blood pressure depends on the strength of the heartbeat, the elasticity of the arterial walls, and the resistance in the capillaries.

At the **age of 20**, the average values are **120 mm of mercury (mm Hg) systolic** and **80 mm Hg diastolic** blood pressure. Under certain circumstances, blood pressure decreases (hypotension) or increases (hypertension).

Memorize	M!
Hypotension refers to chronic blood pressure values below 105/60 mm Hg.	

This is a disturbance in the circulatory regulation, caused by insufficient strength in the heart, blood loss, or experience of shock in acute hypotonia.

Low blood pressure with tendency to circulatory insufficiency is less dangerous than high blood pressure. Hypotension occurs both in younger and older persons.

The typical manifestations of this disease are triggered by insufficient circulation, especially in the brain.

11.2.1 Symptoms

- Low blood pressure in the seated or lying position.
- Reduced physical and mental productivity.
- Fatigue.
- Exhaustion.
- Blackout, dizziness, and fainting.
- Subjective coldness in the limbs, tinnitus, sleep disturbances, irritability.

11.2.2 Suggested Therapy

Most patients do not require medicinal therapy.

Treatment with cupping leads to better circulation and lessens annoying symptoms (▶ Fig. 11.3).

11.2.3 Supplemental Therapy

- **Homeopathy.** In low blood pressure, the patient's general constitution is decisive. Nevertheless, the patient suffers from occasional episodes of fainting or collapse, which require a rapid response. You should therefore familiarize yourself well with collapse remedies. Remedy selection on the basis of constitutional aspects.
- **Phytotherapy.** Strengthening the heart muscle with *hawthorn preparations.*

11.2.4 Alternating Therapy

- **Neural therapy.** Quaddle therapy with local anesthetics paravertebral in the heart segment.
- **Physical therapy.** Kneipp affusions. *Physical activity.*

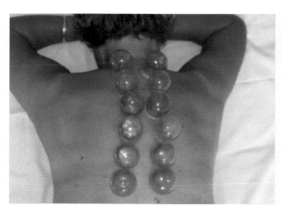

Fig. 11.3 Dry cupping bilaterally along the thoracic vertebrae; alternating with cupping massage.

11.3 High Blood Pressure (Hypertension)

Hypertension refers to a consistent increase (measuring the blood pressure two times daily for a week) in systolic blood pressure above 140 mm Hg and/or diastolic blood pressure above 90 mm Hg. Even if only the systolic blood pressure is elevated, this must be judged as a pathological change.

Upper threshold for normal blood pressure values in children is 115/ 75 mm Hg, from the age of 65, 160/90 mm Hg.

Chronic hypertension mostly results from disorders of the kidneys, the vascular system, or the heart, or of disturbances in internal secretions. In addition, nervous disturbances and chronic overfatigue or overexertion serve as contributing factors. Finally, poisoning and certain heart valve disorders can serve as possible causes of hypertension.

11.3.1 Symptoms

- Without organ complications, no or non-specific symptoms, as a result of which hypertension is often a *coincidental finding.*
- Headache, especially at night.
- Reduced productivity, dizziness, nosebleed, tinnitus, sudden deafness, orthostatic dysregulation.
- Sleep disturbances, especially difficulty falling asleep.
- Tendency to shortness of breath and palpitations.
- In the advanced stage, angina pectoris, chronic coronary insufficiency, neurological, renal, or ocular disturbances.

11.3.2 Suggested Therapy

The aim of cupping therapy in hypertension is to reduce, delay, or improve organ complications, as well as to reduce the dosage of antihypertensive drugs.

Hypertension should be treated in intervals of 2 to 4 weeks if needed.

Note

Treatment with wet cupping can be equated with bloodletting, but can often obtain better results (▶ Fig. 11.4). When withdrawing larger amounts of blood (ca. 300 mL), the elevated blood pressure drops, which often persists for several days or even longer.

Memorize   M!

Do not use wet cupping on patients who *simultaneously* suffer from arrhythmia and coronary insufficiency.

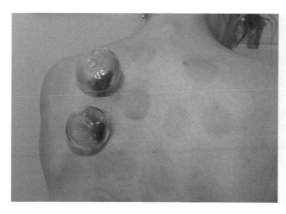

Fig. 11.4 Wet cupping next to the second to fourth thoracic vertebra—on the left side in segments C8–T3.

11.3.3 Supplemental Therapy

- Lowering the blood pressure with **medication**.
- **Homeopathy**. In patients with high blood pressure, the results of homeopathy vary. The different root conditions are decisive for the choice of remedies, if we want to obtain a thorough recovery. The external physical appearance, such as redness and paleness or obesity and emaciation, is already an important indicator of differences and can be the first step leading to differentiation in the choice of remedy.
- **Phytotherapy**. Plant-based antihypertensive drugs like extracts of *Rauwolfia vomitoria,* mistletoe preparations, hawthorn preparations.

11.3.4 Alternating Therapy

- **Neural therapy**. Quaddle therapy with local anesthetics precardial and paravertebral in the heart segment.
- **Physical therapy**. General relaxation and vegetative adjustment.

12 Digestive Organs

12.1 Gastric Catarrh (Gastritis)

Functional disorders of the epigastrium like dyspepsia and stomach spasms are very common. In addition, chronic inflammatory changes in the mucous membranes of the stomach are not rare either. Gastritis refers to an inflammation of the stomach, especially of the gastric mucosa. **Acute gastritis** arises mostly as the result of improper diet, especially excessive alcohol consumption, or less commonly as an accompanying symptom of infectious diseases or kidney failure.

Chronic gastritis always occurs when acute gastritis has not been cured properly. It diffusely affects the entire mucosa of the stomach and can arise as an independent disease, but also as an accompanying symptom of stomach ulcers, carcinomas or diseases of the liver, bile ducts, pancreas, and intestine.

Research has confirmed worldwide by now that type B chronic gastritis (antral gastritis) is triggered by colonization with *Helicobacter pylori*. This bacteria is an important pathogenic factor in the formation of ventricular and duodenal ulcers. Its significance as a high risk factor in stomach carcinomas is under discussion.

12.1.1 Symptoms

- Pressure and feeling of fullness in the upper abdomen, mostly after meals (ulcer-type complaints).
- Nausea.
- Food intolerance.
- Heartburn, frequent belching.
- Pressure in the area of the heart.
- Flatulence.
- Coated tongue.

The symptoms occur in alternation and are aggravated by bad eating habits, for example, hasty eating, substance abuse, medications, but also job-related or social pressures, psychological conflict situations, stress, neuroses, and depression. Allergic factors can also play a certain aggravating role.

12.1.2 Suggested Therapy

With evidence of *Helicobacter pylori*, combined treatment with chemotherapeutic drugs eliminates these bacteria completely and permanently. In patients with functional upper abdominal complaints, the numerous "mucosal protective agents" do bring symptomatic relief, but are not sufficient as cure.

> **Note**
>
> After ruling out organic stomach disease, the treatment of under- and over-acidification of gastric juices, of stomach spasms, and dyspepsia shows a good success rate when the suction cups are placed in the appropriate segments and in the solar plexus (▶ Fig. 12.1, ▶ Fig. 12.2, ▶ Fig. 12.3).

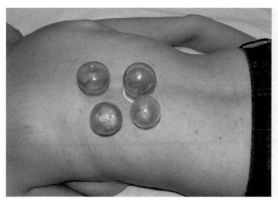

Fig. 12.1 Dry cupping on the left side of the back in segments T2–T9, especially in areas of painful points; potentially also in segment C3.

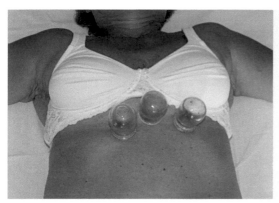

Fig. 12.2 Dry cupping in the solar plexus.

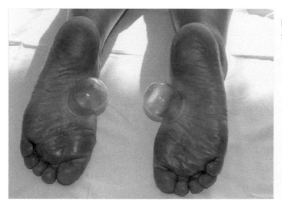

Fig. 12.3 Dry cupping on the stomach-foot reflex zone.

The following formula has proven effective:

Every week, carry out **three cupping treatments**, to a total of **15 treatments**. Follow up with treatments in **2-week intervals**, to a total of **12 treatments**. After this, you can carry out further cupping treatments **once a month** for a certain period of time, depending on success.

12.1.3 Supplemental Therapy

- One of the most important therapeutic measures is to **soothe the patient** and explain the pathophysiological connections. Patients often experience fear of cancer.
- **Homeopathy.** Gastritis responds reliably to homeopathic treatment. In the treatment of acute gastritis, we primarily take the cause of the disorder into consideration, in addition to the symptoms. Options are organotropic, but also constitutional remedies.
- **Phytotherapy.** Tea mixtures or patent preparations, according to syndrome (carminatives, spasmolytics, antiphlogistics, sedatives, bitters).
- **Dietetics.** Patients should avoid foods that they believe to trigger symptoms.

12.1.4 Alternating Therapy

- **Neural therapy.** Subcutaneous injections with a neural drug above the solar plexus and in Head's zones on the back.
- **Baunscheidt therapy.** Above cutivisceral reflexes.

12.2 Acute and Chronic Pancreatitis

We distinguish between two forms of pancreatitis, namely **acute-reversible** and **chronic-progressive.** Both forms are accompanied by pain and functional disturbances of varying intensity, but their causes differ.

Acute pancreatitis arises mostly after infectious disease, after diseases of the bile ducts, stomach, or intestine, or through intoxication or medications.

The causes of **chronic pancreatitis** are alcoholism and chronic inflammations of the stomach, intestine, and bile ducts; psychological traumas and allergies also need to be considered.

12.2.1 Symptoms

- In the acute stage, temperature of 38–39°C (102–104°F).
- Violent pain with sudden onset in the upper abdomen, predominantly on the left, aggravated in the shape of a half belt by movement.
- Cold sweat, nausea, and constipation as a result of intestinal atonia.
- In severe cases, redness of the face and typical drawn-up legs.
- In chronic forms, upper abdominal symptoms generally 2–3 hours after meals, increasing in the evening; pain not always on the left side.
- Belching, diarrhea, flatulence, aversion to fat, intolerances (to raw fruit, yeasted cake, sweets, and coffee), but very variable.
- Emaciation, delayed adaptation to darkness.

12.2.2 Suggested Therapy

A majority of our patients complain of pancreatic symptoms. Advanced pancreatitis not only results in impaired exocrine function, but occasionally also in symptoms of limited endocrine functions.

Memorize	M!
Acute pancreatitis is a medical emergency and must be treated in a hospital.	

In *chronic pancreatitis* or *secretory pancreatic insufficiency,* cupping is recommended after completed examinations and diagnosis (▶ Fig. 12.4 and ▶ Fig. 12.5).

Maintain intervals of 3 days over 6 weeks. Afterwards, due to the chronicity and unpredictability, treat over a longer period of time once per month after symptoms have subsided.

12.2.3 Supplemental Therapy

- **Dietetics.** Maintain easily digestible diet.
- **Homeopathy.** Diseases of the pancreas respond well to homeopathic treatment, if treatable. The number of possible remedies, however, is limited.

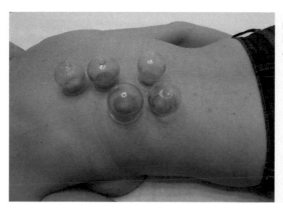

Fig. 12.4 Dry cupping on the back in segments T2-L1, especially in the areas of tender points.

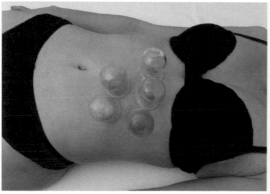

Fig. 12.5 Dry cupping on the upper abdomen on the left side.

- **Phytotherapy.** Swedish bitters three times a day, one teaspoon in an herbal tea of yarrow and marigold. Harongan as patent medicine.
- In pancreatic insufficiency, **enzyme substitution**.

12.2.4 Alternating Therapy

- **Neural therapy.** Quaddle therapy with local anesthetics on the upper abdomen and paravertebral in segments **T7–L1**.

12.3 Liver Disorders

The liver is an organ that switches between two organ systems—the digestive system and the circulatory system. Whenever there is a functional disturbance in one of the systems, sooner or later we are also bound to see disturbances in the liver. Conversely: if the liver is diseased, disorders of the stomach, intestine, and circulatory system result, especially heart problems.

Diseases of the liver are widespread and quite malicious. The patient initially has no complaints for a while because the liver itself does not hurt. Signs of the disease arise only in advanced stages. Because arising complaints are often atypical, it is not always easy to recognize liver disease. Nausea and a feeling of pressure in the upper abdomen first suggest stomach and/or intestinal disorders.

The most well-known symptom is **jaundice**, which can, however, also arise as a secondary symptom of diseases, for example, of the gallbladder, pancreas, or heart, or as a concomitant sign of infections (e.g., Weil disease).

12.3.1 Symptoms

Acute and Chronic Hepatitis

Acute hepatitis is a viral infection, either in the framework of a generalized infection or of an infection limited to the liver. **Chronic hepatitis** develops from the acute form, especially when acute hepatitis is unrecognized and not treated in time. Both forms manifest with the following symptoms:

- In the acute stage, jaundice, beer-brown coloration of urine, fatigue, digestive problems.
- The liver is often enlarged.
- The chronic stage corresponds to acute hepatitis, with the difference that jaundice, liver swelling, and impaired liver functions last longer when they arise.

Liver Cirrhosis

Liver cirrhosis can develop from an uncured case of acute or chronic hepatitis, but also as a result of chronic cholangitis, alcoholism, or persistent malnutrition. The following symptoms are indicative:

- Pressure in the upper abdomen.
- Lack of appetite.
- Nausea.
- Flatulence.

- Depressed mood.
- Fatigue.
- Intolerance to fat.
- Certain signs on the skin (spider nevi, pelmar erythema).

Liver Congestion

Liver congestion arises as a result of heart disease or disturbed blood circulation in the lung. It manifests in the following symptoms:
- Gastrointestinal complaints as a result of liver distention.
- Headache and exhaustion.
- Functional disturbances in the liver are further aggravated by certain medications. Therefore, naturopathic treatments should be given priority in the treatment of liver disorders.

12.3.2 Suggested Therapy

In liver disorders of all types and in every stage, treatment with cupping is recommended as *basic treatment,* because it increases the regenerative capacity of the liver (▶ Fig. 12.6 and ▶ Fig. 12.7).

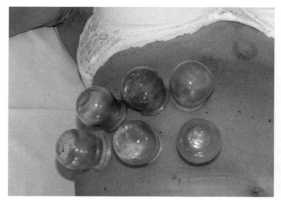

Fig. 12.6 Dry cupping on the upper abdomen on the right side.

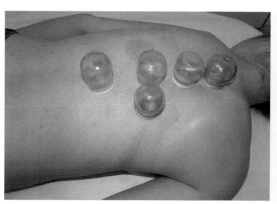

Fig. 12.7 Dry cupping on the back in the liver and gallbladder segments T2–T12, possibly also in segments C4–C6, especially on tender points.

Initially **two to three treatments per week**, to a **total of 12 treatments**. Afterwards, carry out **12 treatments in intervals of 14–21 days**. Subsequently, over a long period of time, **once a month**.

> **Note**
>
> Wet cupping: on the right side in segments T2-T8.

12.3.3 Supplemental Therapy

- **Phytotherapy.** Phytotherapy plays an almost leading role in liver disease because tea infusions or patent preparations assist with a faster detoxification of the liver. Herbal teas or preparations that promote bile flow and diuresis regulate digestion, strengthen the heart and circulation.
- **Dietetics.** The diet should be easy to digest and rich in carbohydrates, protein, and vitamins. Fat from beef, pork, and mutton should be avoided. And in hepatitis, food should be low in protein and fat.
- **Oxygen therapy.** Liver disorders respond particularly well to treatment with oxygen.

12.3.4 Alternating Therapy

- **Homeopathy.** In these diseases, homeopathic remedies can be surprisingly effective, but only with proper diagnosis and selection of remedies. In this area in particular, the right choice is not easy because of the large number of indicated remedies. Liver disorders respond well to organotropic and functiotropic therapy, in which case it often makes sense to find a constitutional remedy.
- **Physical therapy.** Warmth, moist compresses in the area of the liver.
- **Autourine therapy.** An application of autourine therapy makes sense (drinking one's urine; injections).
- **Autohemotherapy.** An application of autologous blood is recommended because it further increases the regenerative capacity of the liver.

12.4 Disorders of the Gallbladder and Bile Ducts

Almost 70% of all humans experience problems in the gallbladder or bile ducts during their lives. The extent of resulting complaints varies considerably and depends on whether the disease is acute or chronic. The cause of **inflammatory disorders** in the area of the gallbladder is often found in an invasion of infectious germs from the intestine or via the bloodstream.

Gallstones, on the other hand, result from the formation of crystals from the substances cholesterol, calcium carbonate, bilirubin, or protein, which are present in the bile and collect in the form of a stone in the gallbladder.

Dyskinesia of the gallbladder and bile ducts is a functional disorder, mostly in the context of vegetative dystonia, without any organic cause.

Cholestasis syndrome—bile congestion results from insufficient or lacking flow of bile to the intestine.

A disorder in the gallbladder is also always a generalized disorder, especially a digestive disturbance. In this context, it is irrelevant whether we are dealing with an inflammation, stone formation, or spasm of the bile ducts. To avoid later effects, we must treat acute and chronic disorders of the gallbladder and bile ducts with great thoroughness.

12.4.1 Symptoms

The most common symptoms of biliary disorders are:
- Common symptoms of hepatic disorders are pain in the right upper abdomen, which can increase to the point of hepatic colic.
- Nausea and fat intolerance.
- Fever and shivering fits point to inflammation of gallbladder or bile ducts.
- An important symptom is obstructive jaundice.
- Severe itching suggests cholestasis.

Memorize	M!
Disorders like empyema or calculous obstruction must obviously be managed with surgical treatment, which must not be delayed. Segmentally bound chronic bilious complaints, on the other hand, can be visibly alleviated or even cured through the segments.	

12.4.2 Suggested Therapy

It has already been mentioned that liver disorders respond well to cupping treatment. Cupping is also recommended in chronic, recurrent disorders in the area of the bile ducts (▶ Fig. 12.8).

The formula is identical to that in the discussion of liver disease (see section 12.3.2).

Note
See ▶ Fig. 12.6: Dry cupping in the upper abdomen on the right side. Wet cupping: on the right side in segments T2–T8.

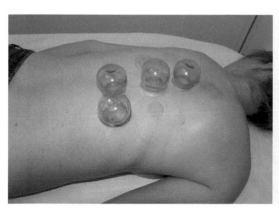

Fig. 12.8 Dry cupping in the gallbladder and liver segments on the right side, T2–T12, also often segment C4, especially in the area of tender points.

12.4.3 Supplemental Therapy

- **Homeopathy.** Here, selecting indicated remedies is not easy either because most homeopathic remedies affect both the liver and the gallbladder. Since gallbladder and liver form a close functional unit, separating the proven remedies would be artificial.
- **Phytotherapy.** In cases of bile congestion where no blockage of the bile ducts is present, to promote bile flow. Tea infusions or patent phytopreparations that contain peppermint, milk thistle, greater celandine, artichokes, and curcuma. Coarsely ground flaxseed mixed in water to regulate digestion.
- **Dietetics.** This is the **most important supplemental measure.** Avoid: deep-fried foods, coffee, legumes, and cabbages, as well as iced drinks.
- **Physical therapy.** Heat applications on the upper abdomen are experienced as very comfortable.

12.4.4 Alternating Therapy

- **Neural therapy.** Quaddle therapy with local anesthetics in the upper abdomen, especially on the right side. Paravertebral on the right side, segments **T5–T12.** Especially *tender points.*
- **Acupuncture.** Causal therapy.
- **Autohemotherapy.** An application of autohemotherapy makes sense.

12.5 Intestinal Disorders

The vital functions of the intestine can be disrupted by multiple diseases that cause changes in the intestinal mucosa.

With the exception of disorders of the straight intestine, ileus, and appendicitis, most intestinal disorders manifest in disturbed *motility* (diarrhea, constipation) and *secretion* (increased amounts of water, electrolytes, phlegm, and protein in the stool), in *increased gas* (meteorism), in *sensitivity* (pain), as well as in the appearance of *pathogenic elements* (blood, pus) and undigested food particles *in the stool.* In addition, disease of the intestinal mucosa influences the *immune system* negatively. As a result, we see weakened resistance and increased frequency of other disorders.

Memorize	M!

Intestinal Inflammation (Enteritis) is a non-ulcerous, usually acute inflammation of the small intestinal mucosa.

In most cases, this disease is caused by *infection* with typhoid, paratyphoid, or enteritis bacteria. Consumption of spoiled food that has been colonized by bacteria from the by-products of decay is also a common cause of intestinal inflammation. In addition, alcohol and chemical poisoning, abuse of laxatives, allergies, helminthiasis, fermentation and putrefaction dyspepsia, and so on.

12.5.1 Symptoms

Acute enteritis begins with sudden onset of diarrhea, in conjunction with spasmodic stomachache:

- Occasionally fever, vomiting, lassitude, coated tongue, as well as substantial thirst.
- The stomach is sensitive to pressure.

In addition to allergies, dysfunctions of the endocrine glands, and lack of vitamins, the key factor responsible for the development of chronic enteritis is very often laxative abuse. Laxatives are substances that irritate the intestinal mucosa. They provoke a mild inflammation and thereby develop their laxative action.

A chronically inflamed intestine is the breeding ground of dangerous bacterial infections. Incidentally, the small intestine rarely develops an inflammation in isolation; generally, the stomach and large intestine are also affected.

Chronic enteritis is associated with the following symptoms:
• Diarrhea (liquid, sometimes mushy).
• Increased gas formation and intestinal noises, sensitivity to pressure.

12.5.2 Suggested Therapy

Persistent diarrhea causes the body to lose nutrients. Chronic intestinal inflammation frequently also leads to disturbed absorption. The result is lack of protein, carbohydrates, fat, electrolytes, water, and vitamins. This has a detrimental effect on all organs. Treatment therefore has the following goals:
• Eliminating the cause.
• Calming the inflamed intestine.
• Replacing the lost nutrients.

In intestinal disease, treatment attempts with cupping are indicated in every case (► Fig. 12.9, ► Fig. 12.10, ► Fig. 12.11):

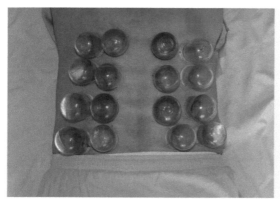

Fig. 12.9 Dry cupping in segments T5-L3 on both sides; also possibly in the reflex zone for the diaphragm.

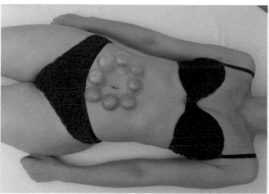

Fig. 12.10 Dry cupping around the navel.

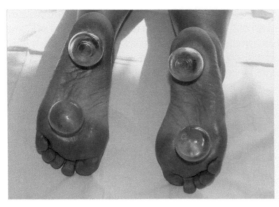

Fig. 12.11 Dry cupping on the foot reflex zones: solar plexus and pelvic organs.

- **Acute stage:** first to third day, **one treatment daily**. From the fourth day on, only **one treatment every third or fifth day** until the complete disappearance of the complaints.
- **Chronic stage**: carry out one treatment every 5 days, to a total of 12–15 treatments.

12.5.3 Supplemental Therapy

- In bacterial infections, **antibiotics** and **bedrest.**
- **Phytotherapy.** In the acute stage, it is helpful to initiate treatment by thoroughly purging the bowels (e.g., with castor oil). This purge causes a rapid discharge of harmful substances and thereby a faster elimination of inflammatory changes in the intestinal mucosa. *Acute cases:* chamomile, oak bark, tormentil root, or black tea. *Chronic cases:* mallow, liquorice, nettle, lemon balm, and marigold.
- **Dietetics.** Acute intestinal inflammation is first treated with days of fasting, during which only tea is permitted. **Avoid the following:** all foods that irritate the intestine or overstrain digestion.
- **Vitamins and minerals.** A, D, K, B, sodium, potassium, calcium, iron.

12.5.4 Alternating Therapy

- **Physical therapy.** *Acute:* moist warm compresses around the stomach several times a day.
- **Autohemotherapy.** *Chronic:* potentiated autologous blood is recommended.

12.6 Constipation (Obstipation)

This refers to a functional disturbance of the digestive tract with delayed evacuation of mostly hard stool.

Constipation can be divided into three forms with different causes:

- An **independent condition** that has persisted for years and is often caused by lack of exercise, diet low in roughage, psychological influences, weakened urge to void due to suppression, slack abdominal wall, or certain medications.

- A **consequence** of tumors and strictures of the large intestine and so on. This type of constipation tends to be short-term only. The stool often contains blood and phlegm.
- A **concomitant symptom** of fever, pregnancy, nephrolithiasis, cholelithiasis, endocrine disturbances (hypothyroidism), vegetative dystonia, longer bedrest, change of residence, and so on.

12.6.1 Symptoms

- Abdominal fullness, missing urge to evacuate the rectum, lack of appetite, belching.
- Formation of gas with increased flatulence.
- Often headache and dizziness, exhaustion.
- Short-lasting spasms that diminish after bowel movements.

12.6.2 Suggested Therapy

Eliminate the cause:
- Regulate the activity of the intestine with sufficient supply of fluids, physical exercise, and a set time for daily bowel movements that the body gets used to.
- Laxative tea only in acute cases and only for a short period of time, because even plant-based laxatives can cause dependency and harm the intestine. In this disease, we must carry out a treatment that is tailored completely to the patient, in accordance with the stage and duration of the disorder (▶ Fig. 12.12).

> **Note**
>
> See ▶ Fig. 12.9: Dry cupping in segments T5-L3 on both sides.

12.6.3 Supplemental Therapy

- **Phytotherapy.** Several times a day, ingest one heaped teaspoon of coarsely ground flaxseed, mixed into a glass of lukewarm water (stimulating peristalsis).

12.6.4 Alternating Therapy

Neural therapy. Quaddle therapy with local anesthetics over the entire course of the colon and in segments **T10-L3**, possibly also segment **C4**.

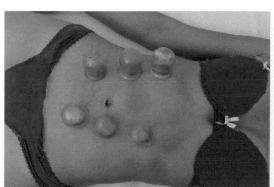

Fig. 12.12 Dry cupping over the ascending and descending colon, possibly also over the entire course of the colon (large intestine).

13 Locomotor System

13.1 Rheumatic Disorders

"Rheumatism" is a collective term for diseases that affect particularly the joints and ligaments of the limbs, the spinal column, tendons, connective tissue, and muscle, but also the internal organs. A typical example is *acute rheumatic fever,* which can lead not only to polyarthritis, but also to heart or kidney disease.

Note

Rheumatic diseases are today categorized in the following groups:
- **Inflammatory rheumatism:**
  - Acute rheumatoid arthritis (rheumatic fever).
  - Chronic rheumatoid arthritis (articular rheumatism).
  - Bechterew disease (ankylosing spondylitis).
- **Degenerative, non-inflammatory rheumatism:**
  - Arthrosis.
  - Spondylosis and osteochondrosis.
- **Soft tissue rheumatism:**
  - This includes partly inflammatory, partly degenerative processes that affect not the joints but the muscles, connective tissue, synovial bursa, tendon sheaths, and nerves.

Rheumatology distinguishes between two different types of pain, namely mechanical pain and inflammatory pain.

Mechanical pain generally appears during or after physical exertion, abates during rest, and completely disappears overnight. If stiffness does occur in the morning, it is very short and lasts a few minutes at most.

In contrast, **inflammatory pain** occurs also when the patient is resting. Generally, it flares up during the second half of the night and in some cases becomes so severe toward the morning that it awakens the patient. Inflammatory pain tends to be accompanied by **ankylosis.** This early-morning stiffness is persistent and painful, possibly lasting for more than half an hour. In contrast, ankylosis in conjunction with arthrosis generally lasts only a few minutes.

13.1.1 Symptoms

Acute Rheumatic Fever

Acute rheumatoid arthritis refers to a hypersensitive reaction (allergy) to pathogens, most commonly *streptococcus* bacteria. This condition manifests in sudden fever of up to 40°C (104°F) in conjunction with very painful redness and swelling in the joints; the large and medium-sized joints (joints of the knees, feet, shoulders, elbows, and hands) are particularly affected.

A typical characteristic of this disease is that it *wanders,* from one joint to another. Also typical is profuse sweating. The sweat has a characteristic sour odor.

Shortly before the onset of acute rheumatoid arthritis, the patient often suffers from tonsillitis or catarrh of the nose, throat, and bronchial tubes. This disease most frequently affects children and young adults, but especially school children.

> **Cave**
>
> Because of the severity of the disease and the danger of secondary developments, especially of rheumatic carditis, hospitalization is often necessary.

Inflammatory Chronic Rheumatoid Arthritis (Articular Rheumatism)

Chronic rheumatoid arthritis is also inflammatory, but not caused by pathogens. The cause is unknown. Because the chronic inflammation is self-perpetuating and hence does not heal, autoimmune processes have been suspected as formative. The disease can occur in all ages, but predominantly between the ages of 25 and 50, and affects women at three times the rate as men.

- As a rule, latent disease onset with joint problems that are at first undefined, such as stiffness in the finger and hand joints, especially in the morning after waking.
- Later, pain and swelling develops in the joints. The small joints on the hands and feet are involved first.
- In more advanced stages of the disease, the larger joints and parts of the cervical spinal column are also affected. Sooner or later, deformities develop in the hands and feet.
- Deterioration of general health, such as fatigue, exhaustion, lack of appetite, weight loss, abnormal sweating and mild anemia, sometimes slightly elevated body temperature.

Degenerative Rheumatoid Arthritis (Arthrosis)

Arthrosis is not an inflammatory disorder, but a degenerative joint disease that affects primarily the joint cartilage. The cause of arthrosis is a disproportion between the load and load-bearing capacity of the joint surfaces. In this process, the following factors play a role amongst others:

- Congenital or injury-related malposition of the joints.
- Congenital weakness of the cartilage tissue.
- Previous joint inflammations.
- Hormonal influences.
- Excessive weight.
- Strain.

The disease is relatively widespread. It occurs mostly after the age of 40 and is slightly more common in women than in men.

In principle, it can affect any joint, but is most common in the load-bearing joints such as the knee, hip, and foot joints, and the small joints of the lumbar spinal column, followed by the shoulder, elbow, and hand joints.

- The first indications of arthrosis are *stiffness* and *a feeling of tension* after longer rest periods.

- Pain in arthrosis is predominantly *mechanical* pain during starting or warm-up that decreases with further movement is typical. Continuous strain, however, induces repeated pain.
- As the clinical picture of arthrosis progresses, bony enlargements may form in the joints, and you may hear grinding or crackling noises. The motility of the joints is limited due to pain.
- Continuous sparing of the joint increases the danger of articular stiffness due to limited movement.
- Furthermore, lack of movement leads to poor circulation in the joint capsule and therefore to additional impaired nutrition in the already damaged cartilage.

13.1.2 Suggested Therapy

The treatment of rheumatic disorders with cupping (▶ Fig. 13.1, ▶ Fig. 13.2, ▶ Fig. 13.3, ▶ Fig. 13.4, ▶ Fig. 13.5, ▶ Fig. 13.6) pursues two goals:
- Eliminating the inflammatory symptoms and pain.
- Influencing metabolism, to slow down the decline in degenerative diseases and finally reach stabilization.

By stimulating circulation, cupping loosens the connective tissue, releases tension, and accelerates metabolism. It also relieves the manifestations of inflammation, and therefore the pain.

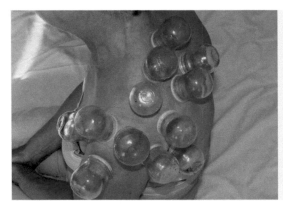

Fig. 13.1 Painful shoulder stiffness (periarthritis of the shoulder). Dry cupping around the diseased joint, in the area of the pain.

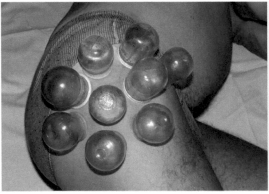

Fig. 13.2 Chronic inflammation of the hip joint (cox arthrosis). Dry cupping around the diseased joint, in the area of the pain.

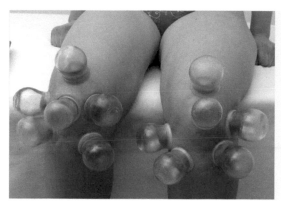

Fig. 13.3 Inflammation of the knee joint (osteoarthritis). Dry cupping around the diseased joint.

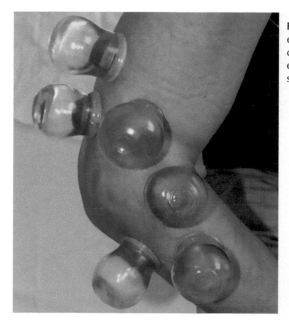

Fig. 13.4 Elbow pain (tennis elbow). Dry cupping around the diseased joint. Application on the elbow joint is only possible with small or medium-sized cups.

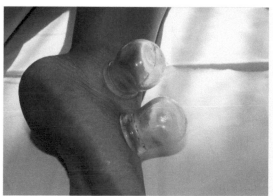

Fig. 13.5 Pain in the ankle joints. Dry cupping around the joint.

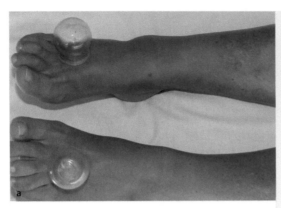

Fig. 13.6 (a, b) Pain in the ankle joints. Dry cupping on painful locations.

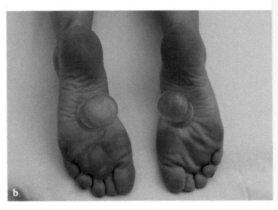

Note

Even major changes can be achieved through treatment, in spite of the fact that improvement often occurs very slowly.

Treatment must be repeated for a longer period of time in intervals of initially **2–4 days**, and afterwards of **8–14 days**, until the goal is reached.

Rubbing ointment on the treated skin areas prior to cupping increases the effect.

Memorize M!

If the patient is suffering from lymphatic congestion in the knee joint, especially in a latent state, it is possible that the cups fall off right after they have been applied for the first treatment. You can see from the steamed up cupping glasses that the lymphatic fluid has been put in motion. With patience, you can achieve good or even excellent treatment results.

13.1.3 Supplemental Therapy

Homeopathy. For the rheumatic class of disorders, homeopathy offers a good option for treatment. Nevertheless, a successful homeopathic treatment requires patience from both the therapist and the patient. Remedies must be selected strictly according to individual symptoms.

13.1.4 Alternating Therapy

- **Neural therapy.** Quaddle therapy with local anesthetics above painful joints.
- **Physical therapy.** Depending on tolerance: heat or cold applications.
- **Acupuncture.** Causal therapy.

13.2 Spondylitis

Spondylitis refers to a chronic inflammatory rheumatoid disease that begins with an inflammation of the iliosacral joints and then progressively affects different sections of the spinal column in an ascending order. The supporting tendons and ligaments calcify, which results in increasing stiffness. The cause is still unknown.

> **Note**
>
> The disease is not at all rare. It presents predominantly in men and occurs mostly between the age of 20 and 30.

13.2.1 Symptoms

- Uncharacteristic pain in the joints and back, as well as iritis (inflammation of the iris).
- Later, progressive rigidity of the spinal column, which simultaneously becomes increasingly round in the area of the chest.
- In serious cases, gazing straight forward becomes difficult.
- The disease can also spread to other joints.
- Increasing shortness of breath.
- In a small proportion of patients, vision disturbances.

13.2.2 Suggested Therapy

Like rheumatic and arthritic disorders, spondylitis is also one of the indications for *dry* cupping treatment. The cups stimulate circulation, release tension, loosen the connective tissue, and accelerate metabolism (▶ Fig. 13.7).

> **Note**
>
> Treatments occur **twice a week**, for a period of **2 months**. Following this, one treatment **every 4 weeks** for an extended period of time.

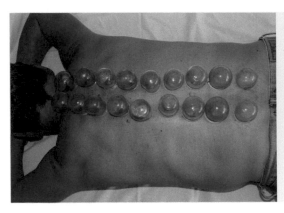

Fig. 13.7 Dry cupping bilaterally along the spinal column, alternating with cupping massage.

13.2.3 Supplemental Therapy

- **Homeopathy.** The states of pure pain in this disease do not yet allow a proper selection of remedies. Rather, the therapist must let him or herself be guided by changes in the spinal column, which lead to the selection of an effective remedy. Organotropic and constitutional treatment offers varied pain relief or slowdown of the advancing process until a complete cure is achieved.
- **Oxygen therapy.** Application of oxygen therapy is useful.

13.2.4 Alternating Therapy

- **Neural therapy.** Quaddle therapy with local anesthetics above painful points.
- **Physical therapy.** Depending on tolerance, heat or cold applications.
- **Baunscheidt therapy.** Paravertebral treatment.
- **Canthardin plasters.** Paravertebral treatment.
- **Acupuncture.** Causal therapy.

13.3 Spondylosis

Spondylosis refers to processes similar to degenerative rheumatoid arthritis. Damage occurs on the vertebral bodies. Spondylosis is most likely to develop in the lower sections of the lumbar and cervical spinal column. Like arthrosis, degenerative changes in the spinal column are extremely widespread. These changes are found primarily in older persons.

13.3.1 Symptoms

- Chronic or recurrent back pain.
- Limited mobility.
- The generative changes in the cervical spinal column occasionally cause pain in the neck, back of the head, shoulder, and arm, as well as sensory disturbances and feelings of weakness in the arm (shoulder-arm syndrome).
- Spondylosis can lead to acute lumbago or slipped disk.

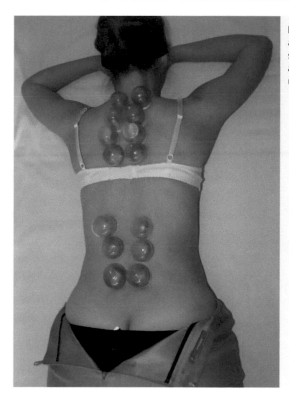

Fig. 13.8 Dry cupping bilaterally along the cervical and/or lumbar spinal column. *Cupping massage* as alternating treatment is always useful.

13.3.2 Suggested Therapy

The application of cupping in diseases of the spinal column can eliminate numerous complaints, including changes in the vertebrae (▶ Fig. 13.8).

Note
Course of treatment as in *spondylitis*.

13.3.3 Supplemental Therapy

- **Homeopathy.** The alleviation of symptoms depends on how far advanced the degenerative changes in the spinal column are. Nevertheless, relief of pain can often still be achieved even in such cases. Selection of remedy in accordance with the constitutional event involved in each case.
- **Oxygen therapy.** Application can be useful.

13.3.4 Alternating Therapy

- **Neural therapy.** Quaddle therapy with local anesthetics into tender points.
- **Physical therapy.** Short-wave radiation and other heat applications.
- **Baunscheidt therapy.** Paravertebral therapy.

- **Cantharidin plasters.** Paravertebral treatment.
- **Acupuncture.** Causal therapy.

13.4 Lumbago

Acute lumbago is the result of pathologic changes in the lumbar spinal column, especially of damage to the intervertebral disks, which leads to irritation of the nerves that supply the muscles of the back. Lumbago has a sudden onset, most commonly after malposture in the back, lifting objects, or carrying loads.

13.4.1 Symptoms

- Severe pain that is aggravated by movement or coughing in the lumbar area, forcing the patient to bend forward in relieve posture.
- Hard, tensed lumbar muscles.
- In slipped disk, pain on the back side of the leg down to the heel.

13.4.2 Suggested Therapy

In this case, success can be attained already **after the first treatment.** If not, repeat treatment **in intervals of 4 days**, until complete absence of complaints is reached (▶ Fig. 13.9 and ▶ Fig. 13.10).

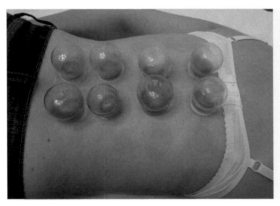

Fig. 13.9 Dry cupping bilaterally along the lumbar spinal column on tender points, in alternation with cupping massage.

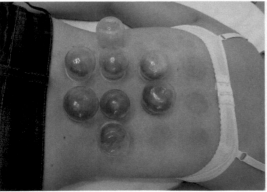

Fig. 13.10 Dry cupping in the area of pain; cupping massage as alternating treatment.

13.4.3 Supplemental Therapy

- **Homeopathy.** Acute lumbago should, with rare exceptions, offer the chance of a "miracle treatment" for the homeopathic therapist. In acute cases, the pain generally subsides quickly after taking organotropic homeopathic remedies. In chronic cases, success depends on the severity of the disease and on the degree of pre-existing spinal column deformations. The number of possible remedies is quite large.
- **Neural therapy.** Depending on the case, quaddle therapy with local anesthetics.

13.4.4 Alternating Therapy

- **Physical therapy.** Peat, mud, or sulfur baths; short-wave radiation and other heat applications.
- **Baunscheidt therapy.** Paravertebral treatment.
- **Canthardin plasters.** Paravertebral treatment.
- **Acupuncture.** Causal therapy.

14 Reproductive Organs

14.1 Female Reproductive Organs

14.1.1 Menstrual Disorders, Inflammations of the Reproductive Organs

All healthy women menstruate during their fertile years. The time between the first and last menstrual period spans ~30–40 years. During this time, typical repeated changes occur in the endometrium and the menstrual period returns regularly, according to a cycle of roughly 4 weeks.

The processes in the female organism by no means always pass without mishaps. Some women experience discomfort when menstruating, suffering from cramps, headache, and other symptoms.

The female menstrual cycle is one of the best examples for the complicated interrelationships between different hormones. The entire endocrine system is involved. Furthermore, other organ systems must also function correctly to ensure that the cycles proceed normally. Diseases of the thyroid gland, for example, cause menstrual irregularities or even a complete absence of menstruation. The activity of the ovaries, which determines menstrual bleeding, is not always stable. Stress, mental strain, even just a change of surroundings or jobs, extremely high or low weight, certain medications, and infections or other diseases are only some of the many factors that can disrupt a woman's reproductive cycle.

The strength and duration of menstruation, but also the type of pain, provide clues about both healthy as well as disturbed activities of the female organs.

> **Note**
>
> Any unresolved menstrual irregularity must be examined by a specialist.

Inflammatory diseases of the ovaries and uterus are also responsible for menstrual irregularities. The causes for these diseases are mostly infections that ascend from the vagina upward, and in addition, for the uterus, inflammations that descend from the fallopian tubes and ovaries.

Symptoms

- Feeling of pressure in the lower abdomen, labor-like pain, menstrual disorders.
- Often fever, occasionally with sudden attacks of shivering.
- After the cause has been determined, cupping can lead to fast results, also in combination with measures from conventional Western medicine.

Suggested Therapy

Cupping can be applied with good results in all gynecological diseases listed next (▶ Fig. 14.1, ▶ Fig. 14.2, ▶ Fig. 14.3, ▶ Fig. 14.4).

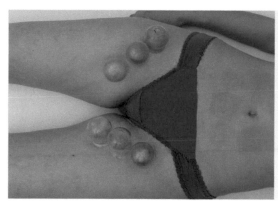

Fig. 14.1 Dry cupping in the groin over Head's zone for the uterus and adnexa.

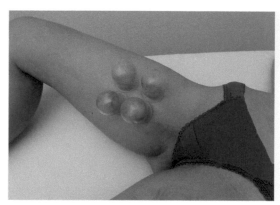

Fig. 14.2 Dry cupping on the inside of the thigh. According to acupuncture theory, connections exist to the inflamed genitalia.

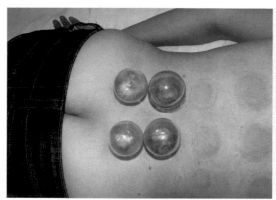

Fig. 14.3 Dry cupping on both sides of the spinal column in segments L1-L5.

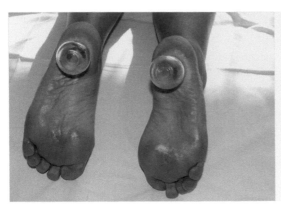

Fig. 14.4 Dry cupping on the foot reflex zones for adnexa (gonads).

- **Adnexitis, endometriosis:**
  - Treatment initially occurs **in intervals of 7 days**, ca. **three treatments**; afterwards, in **intervals of 14 days**, approximately also **three treatments**.
  - Additional measures in consideration of the stage of the disease and the situation of the patient.
- **Amenorrhea, hypermenorrhea, menorrhagia, dysmenorrhea:**
  - In these conditions, continue treatment in intervals of **10 days for 3 months**. Afterwards, treatment depends on the development of the disease.
  - If therapy is continued, keep treating in larger intervals of **3–4 weeks**.

> **Note**
>
> For disorders in the genital area, see ▶ Fig. 14.9: Dry cupping ca. 1.5 cm below the navel.

Supplemental Therapy

- For inflammations, **bedrest** can be useful.
- **Homeopathy.** Homeopathic treatment of any of these diseases generally achieves good results. In these cases, organotropic and functiotropic remedies are indicated, but the therapist must, as so often, choose among a large number of remedies.
- **Physical therapy.** Cold or warm compresses; sitz baths can complement the treatment and accelerate recovery.
- **Phytotherapy.** Extracts that have a sedative and spasmolytic effect (lemon balm, yarrow).

Alternating Therapy

- **Neural therapy.** Quaddle therapy with local anesthetics on top of the ventral Head's zones of the lower abdomen and on top of the sacrum.
- **Autohemotherapy.** Autohemotherapy is indicated.
- **Baunscheidt therapy.** For detoxification and promotion of immune resistance, it can be useful as alternating therapy.

14.1.2 Climacteric Disorders

Menopause, also called "climacteric period," is the stage in a woman's life when ovulation and menstruation cease and hence the years of fertility end.

The biological effect of menopause is a process that extends over 5–10 years, during which the activity of the ovaries drops off and then stops altogether. It is important to remember that a natural menopause, in contrast with a surgically induced one, is not a disease but a biological process that can be divided into three stages:

- Premenopause.
- Menopause.
- Postmenopause.

Menopause can be accompanied by a multiplicity of symptoms that are related to hormonal changes. It varies, however, from woman to woman. Some women barely notice it; others suffer from frequent hot flashes that almost incapacitate them, night sweats, mood swings, depression, irritability, insomnia, poor circulation, cardiac disorders, and other symptoms that point to metabolic disorders and can persist for several years.

Treatment in conventional Western medicine, which replaces the estrogen lacking after menopause, is controversial. Furthermore, some women experience side-effects in this hormone therapy, which manifest in swelling, increased weight, nausea, vomiting, headache, heightened susceptibility to vaginal fungal infections and bleeding, and swollen and tender breasts.

Suggested Therapy

It is important to influence the genital area (▶ Fig. 14.5 and ▶ Fig. 14.6). Two treatments per week are recommended, to a total of **15 cupping treatments**. To stabilize results, follow up with **one cupping treatment in intervals of 3 weeks**. Afterwards, carry out **one treatment per month** if necessary.

> **Note**
>
> See ▶ Fig. 14.3: Dry cupping on both sides of the spinal column in segments **L1–L5** and next to the sacrum.
> In hypertonicity, additionally also wet cupping.

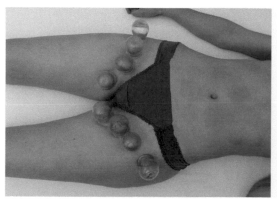

Fig. 14.5 Dry cupping in the groin over the Head's zone for the uterus and adnexa.

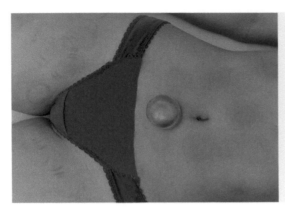

Fig. 14.6 Dry cupping ca. 3 cm below the navel; influencing a disrupted menstrual cycle.

Supplemental Therapy

- **Homeopathy.** The time of menopause affects women in every aspect of their existence. Different symptoms appear in this transitional stage, manifesting on the physical, emotional, and mental level. From a homeopathic perspective, it is not the individual symptom that points to the correct choice of remedies in these disorders, but the potential total of all symptoms. Choice of individual remedies according to homeopathic principles, as important supplemental therapy.
- **Phytotherapy.** For patients with depressed mood swings and nervous irritability, extracts of hypericum, passiflora, or hops. The last of these has a sedative and an estrogenic effect.

Alternating Therapy

- **Neural therapy.** Quaddle therapy with local anesthetics on top of the ventral Head's zones of the lower abdomen and on top of the sacrum.
- **Cantharidin plasters.** Therapy in cases with imminent hypertonicity.
- **Baunscheidt therapy.** Paravertebral treatment in segment L5.
- **Autohemotherapy.** Can be useful.

14.1.3 Sexual Malfunctions in Women

The course of women's sexual lives is not always free of obstacles. On the contrary, it can be disturbed on multiple levels.

The most common malfunctions are caused by psychological strain, as a result of which many women are no longer able to feel the natural sexual urge, let alone sexual climax. These psychologically stressful factors include:
- Unconscious negative attitude toward sexuality as a result of upbringing.
- Fright.
- Uncomfortable sexual experience (sexual abuse).
- Extramarital affairs.

The partner's irresponsible behavior can also trigger sexual malfunctions or even aversion to the partner and extinguish sexual feelings in the woman altogether.

Sexual malfunctions and deviations associated with sexual life include the following:
- Complete lack of desire for sex (libido).
- Absence of the ability to achieve orgasm during sexual intercourse (anorgasmia or frigidity).
- Inability of the woman to orgasm during sexual intercourse at the same time as her partner (dyspareunia).

Dysfunctions of the sexual act and of sexual satisfaction are nowadays found in a surprisingly high percentage of women.

The **complete absence of desire** for sexual contact is pathological and often conditioned by physical factors. Possible causes are:
- Underdevelopment of the genital organs.
- Serious general illness.
- Disorders of the central nervous system.

The **absence of orgasm** is one of the states of sexual inability, similar to impotence in men. The basic difference is that men are unable to have sexual intercourse in the state of sexual impotence, while women (in the state of complete absence of orgasm) with rare exceptions are almost always still able to have sexual intercourse.

Anorgasmia can have physical as well as psychological causes: sensory disorders with a physical basis have causes both in the area of the genitalia, for example, infections, vaginal stricture, and so on, and in serious general diseases, fatigue from one's work or lifestyle, deficient or wrong nutrition, and the effect of certain medicinal drugs.

Because women by nature need more time than men to orgasm, simultaneous satisfaction is not always guaranteed for them. If the man reaches a satisfying climax at the very beginning of sexual intercourse, the fault for this does not lie with the woman, but also with the man. A real deviation exists when the woman requires an unnaturally long period of time to achieve an orgasm.

As a rule, sexual malfunctions appear in conjunction with other indications of vegetative dysregulation, such as:
- Poor circulation.
- Weak concentration.
- Palpitations.

Women who suffer from sexual malfunction require as much affection and understanding as impotent men to reach an unforced and natural, sexually relaxing feeling of sensuality.

After structural causes have been eliminated, repeated cupping can attempt to influence the genitalia and rebalance vegetative dysregulation.

Suggested Therapy

The following formula has proven effective for treatment:

Initially, two to three treatments per week, to a total of **18 treatments**. Afterwards, you can increase intervals between treatments **initially to 2 weeks**, later to **4 weeks**, depending on success.

Treatment example:
- First treatment day: cupping sites as in ▶ Fig. 14.2 and ▶ Fig. 14.9.
- Second treatment day: cupping sites as in ▶ Fig. 14.7 and ▶ Fig. 14.8.
- Third treatment day: as on first day.
- Fourth treatment day: as on second day, and so on.

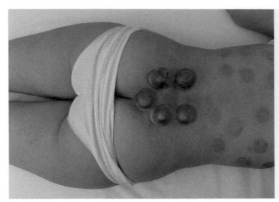

Fig. 14.7 Dry cupping on the sacrum, over the sacral cavities.

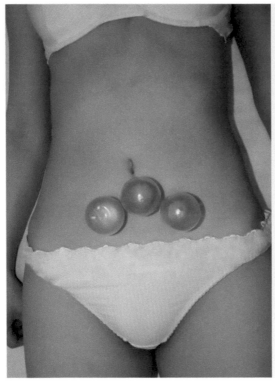

Fig. 14.8 Dry cupping on the lower abdomen, over the bladder region.

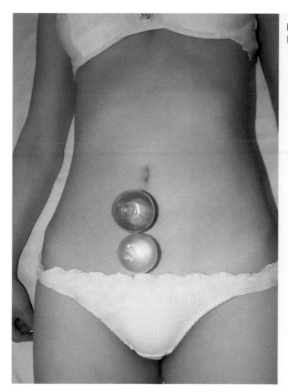

Fig. 14.9 Dry cupping ca. 1.5 cm below the navel.

Note

See ▶ Fig. 14.2: Dry cupping at the inside of the upper thigh.

Supplemental Therapy

- If necessary, **psychotherapy.**
- **Homeopathy.** Sexual malfunctions have many triggers that can manifest in such symptoms as inability, tension, and feelings of guilt. The more closely the chosen homeopathic remedies correspond to the expression of the patient, the faster success will be achieved. Among possible homeopathic remedies, organotropic and constitutional aspects must be taken into consideration.

Alternating Therapy

- **Acupuncture.** Symptomatic treatment.
- **Neural therapy.** Quaddle therapy with local anesthetics on top of Head's zones and the sacrum, also intravenous injections.
- **Physical therapy.** Baths with herbal additives (chestnut, arnica, calamus). Embrocations on top of the sacrum have also proven effective. Strengthening of the entire musculature with **gymnastics**.

14.2 Male Reproductive Organs

14.2.1 Inflammation of the Prostate (Prostatitis)

> **Note**
>
> Infectious diseases of the prostate occur frequently in younger men between the age of 20 and 40.

The development of **acute prostatitis** is most commonly caused by infections that spread primarily from neighboring organs like the kidneys and bladder, urethra and intestines, but also via the blood and lymph vessels after a case of influenza, angina, pneumonia, chronic tonsillitis, and so on.

Chronic prostatitis forms either as a primary or secondary chronic inflammation after an incompletely cured acute prostatitis.

The anatomical position of the prostate favors colonization by germs, as a result of which the prostate turns into a center of bacterial activity (comparable to the teeth or tonsils). Temporarily inactive bacteria that have settled there can be activated at any time by weakened resistance and become the cause of many diseases, especially recurrent urogenital diseases.

Symptoms

- Frequent urge to urinate, pain during urination.
- In advanced stage, urinary retention.
- Pressure at the perineum and feeling of fullness in the straight intestine.
- Pain in the back.
- Aggravation of symptoms after cooling off.

Treatment with antibiotics is lengthy and often not very successful. Remissions are not rare.

> **Memorize**　　　　　　　　　　　　　　　　　　　　　　　　　**M!**
>
> **Venereal diseases require specific antibiotic therapy!**

Suggested Therapy

Treatment with cupping improves circulation and nourishment of the tissue (▸ Fig. 14.10, ▸ Fig. 14.11, ▸ Fig. 14.12).

- **Acute stage:** treatment every 2 days, with a total of **10 treatments**.
- **Chronic stage**: here, we schedule treatments at greater intervals from the start, that is, **one treatment every 5 days**. Nevertheless, you have to continue these for a long time until you can be sure that the condition is cured completely. A total of **15 to 18 treatments.**

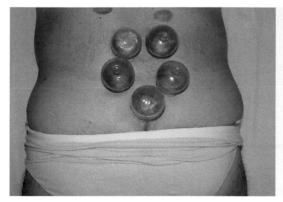

Fig. 14.10 Dry cupping on the sacrum, over the sacral cavities

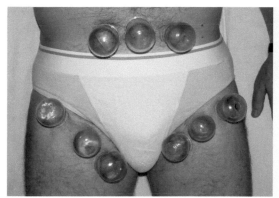

Fig. 14.11 Dry cupping on the lower abdomen and in the groin.

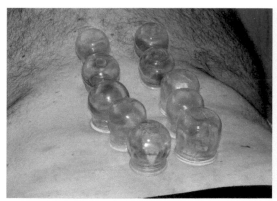

Fig. 14.12 Dry cupping on both sides of the spinal column in segments T11-L5.

Supplemental Therapy

- **Homeopathy.** Homeopathy can successfully treat acute and chronic prostatitis. Therapy requires the doctor to have a lot of experience.
- **Physical therapy.** Warm sitz baths.
- **Phytotherapy.** Extracts with diuretic and tonifying effects (tube curare [homeopathic name: *Pareira Brava*], saw palmetto [*Serenoa repens*]).
- **Dietetics.** Abundant supply of fluids; alcohol and carbonated drinks are prohibited.

Alternating Therapy

- **Neural therapy.** Quaddle therapy with local anesthetics over the sacrum and lower abdomen, over the Head's zones.
- **Baunscheidt therapy.** Over the lumbosacral area.
- **Acupuncture.** According to symptoms.
- **Autohemotherapy.** Achieves satisfying results.

14.2.2 Sexual Malfunctions in Men (Erectile Dysfunction)

Impotence refers to sterility (impotentia generandi) and to inability to develop or maintain an erection in the penis or premature ejaculation (impotentia coeundi) and therefore, in both cases, softening of the penis before sexual intercourse. Hence, this means inability to perform the sexual act (coitus).

Note
When evaluating sexual malfunctions in men, we must, however, take into consideration that male sexual performance gradually declines already from the age of 25 on. From the age of 50 on, potency deteriorates rapidly, both with regards to the sexual urge and to the frequency of intercourse.

Every man can become impotent, but absolute impotence is relatively rare. Physical and psychological conditions can be the reason:
- Psychological inhibitions (may be caused, for example, by an early frightening experience, aversion to a certain female partner, fear of failure, and so on).
- Serious general diseases and states of exhaustion.
- Disorders of the spinal cord and brain.
- Deformed foreskin and urethra.

A more common cause of impotence, however, is *disturbance of the blood supply*. Patients affected with this condition additionally complain of circulatory problems, especially in the lower extremities.

Regardless of what the cause of impotence is, when it exists, it burdens the man considerably. The reason for this is that sexual malfunction is experienced as failure and shameful weakness, which is based on the societal prejudice that manliness is judged by sexual performance. The occurrence of impotence therefore tends to affect a man's self-esteem, and he requires intensive, loving affection, even if he believes himself to be impotent.

Treatment of impotence with *hormone preparations* in an otherwise healthy man is only rarely effective. The same is true for aphrodisiacs, which may be suitable for increasing excitability, but can also have a dangerous effect. In internal overexcitation and excessive fearful psychological tension, psychotherapy or sedatives are most effective.

In cases where the impotence has a physical cause, this must, of course, be eliminated first with the appropriate treatment. If potency is restored after completion of the treatment, we know for sure that no further causes, such as psychological ones, were involved.

Suggested Therapy

Repeated cupping treatments have a favorable effect on the genital organs and their blood supply.

Initially three treatments per week, with a **total of 20 treatments**. Afterwards, you can extend intervals between treatments to **2 weeks, then 3 weeks,** depending on success.

Example of treatment:
- First treatment day: cupping sites as in ► Fig. 14.10 and ► Fig. 14.13.
- Second treatment day: cupping sites as in ► Fig. 14.14 and ► Fig. 14.15.
- Third treatment day: cupping sites as on first day.
- Fourth treatment day: cupping sites as on second day.

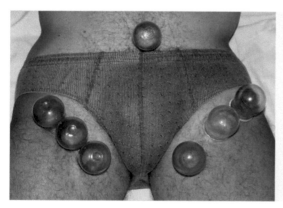

Fig. 14.13 Dry cupping ca. 3 cm below the navel and in the groin.

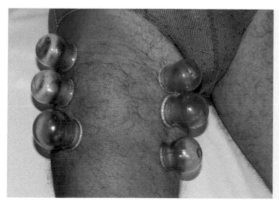

Fig. 14.14 Dry cupping on the inside and outside of the thigh.

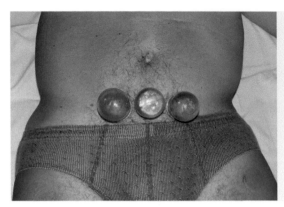

Fig. 14.15 Dry cupping on the lower abdomen, over the bladder region.

Note

See ▶ Fig. 14.10: Dry cupping on the sacrum, over the sacral cavities.

Supplemental Therapy

- **Homeopathy.** Depending on symptoms, the appropriate homeopathic remedies are indicated. When gathering information on the patient's problems, remember that he does not necessarily have to manifest with the complete range of symptoms; often a discrete expression is sufficient indication to make the proper choice of remedy.
- **Phytotherapy.** Tea from calamus root as generally strengthening remedy.

Alternating Therapy

- **Neural therapy.** Quaddle therapy with local anesthetics over the Head's zones and in segments for the reproductive organs.
- **Physical therapy.** Baths with herbal additives (calamus, chestnut, arnica). Embrocations over the sacrum have also proven effective.

15 Urinary Tracts

15.1 Inflammation of the Kidneys (Nephritis, Acute and Chronic)

Acute inflammation of the kidneys in most cases arises suddenly after infectious diseases like angina or scarlet fever, as a complication in which the pathogens reach the kidneys via the blood vessels, or as hypersensitivity to bacteria. This disease primarily affects children and younger adults. The pathological processes take place evenly in the entire kidney tissue.

   Chronic nephritis, on the other hand, refers to a bilateral kidney disorder with chronic inflammatory or scarring changes in the kidney tissue. This disease develops most commonly from an acute kidney inflammation but can also arise *suddenly* without a previous acute stage.

15.1.1 Symptoms

Acute Nephritis

- Generalized symptoms like nausea, lack of appetite, weakness, and headache.
- Occasional pain or dull feeling in the kidney region as well as reduced urination with reddish-brown coloration.
- Elevated temperature.

Chronic Nephritis

- Edemas that occur most frequently or exclusively in the face and hands (backs of the hands).
- Especially typical is early-morning edema in the eyelids and cheeks.
- High blood pressure, weakness, nausea, paleness, itching, and lack of appetite are additional symptoms.
- In the advanced stage, chronic nephritis leads to secondary nephrosclerosis.

Memorize	M!
Chronic nephritis must be taken very seriously and treated resolutely because the advanced stage leads to chronic nephrosclerosis. Additional infections of all types—including respiratory illnesses—must be avoided because they could have an additional negative effect on the diseased kidneys.	

15.1.2 Suggested Therapy

The results of cupping therapy in kidney disease are good (▸ Fig. 15.1). Treatment must be finely tuned to the patient and performed in accordance with the duration and stage of the disease.

   Initially, choose **intervals of 5 days,** with a total of **10 treatments.** Afterwards, continue treatment in **intervals of 14 days,** also approximately **10 treatments.**

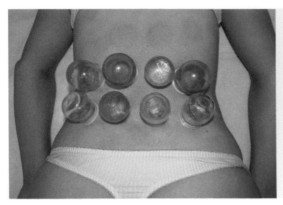

Fig. 15.1 Dry cupping on the back, segments T10–L3. If the urinary bladder is involved, also over the Head's zones for the bladder.

15.1.3 Supplemental Therapy

- **Antibiotics** if necessary.
- **Homeopathy.** Disorders of the kidneys and abducting urinary tracts respond well to homeopathic treatment. In this disease, triggers, state of health, and disposition are interrelated. Treatment of the acute stage is performed with organotropic and functiotropic remedies. For follow-up treatment, select remedies according to constitutional aspects.
- **Phytotherapy.** Herbal teas (horsetail, rupturewort, restharrow, etc.).
- **Physical therapy.** Warm sitz baths with addition of herbal extracts (horsetail).
- **Dietetics.** Sufficient fluid supply, diet with moderately low intake of table salt.

Memorize	M!
Complete withdrawal of sodium, however, can over time be life-threatening.	

15.1.4 Alternating Therapy

- **Neural therapy.** Quaddle therapy with local anesthetics over the associated segments and Head's zones; intravenous injections.
- **Autohemotherapy.** Can be useful.

15.2 Inflammation of the Bladder (Cystitis)

Inflammation of the urinary bladder is a relatively common disease. In this disorder, bacteria settle in the mucous membranes of the bladder, which is connected to other parts of the urinary system. Bacterial infections can either spread from the kidneys downward or from the outside in. Women are more frequently affected because their urethra is much shorter, as a result of which bacteria can more easily travel from the genital area into the urethra. Additional possible causes are getting drenched, cystoscopy, and catheterization.

15.2.1 Symptoms

- Acute cystitis does not engender fever. *Elevated temperature* suggests involvement of the *renal pelvis* or the *prostate gland.*
- Frequent urge to urinate, characteristic pain at the end of urination, weak bleeding.
- The *pain* persists *unchanged day and night.* In contrast, the pain associated with an irritated bladder (cystalgia) lessens at night.

15.2.2 Suggested Therapy

Inflammation of the bladder must be treated resolutely since relapses are common (▶ Fig. 15.2). Treatment is performed according to the following formula: **First, third, and fifth day, one cupping treatment each**. This treatment can be continued for a while if necessary.

> **Note**
>
> See ▶ Fig. 14.15: Dry cupping on the lower abdomen, over the Head's zone for the bladder region.
> If the kidneys are involved, additionally:
> See ▶ Fig. 15.1: Dry cupping on the back, segments T10–L3.

15.2.3 Supplemental Therapy

- If necessary, **antibiotics.**
- **Homeopathy.** Cystitis can generally be controlled well with homeopathic therapy, most of the time without side-effects. Knowing the exact cause facilitates the selection of remedies, which is not easy in this disease because the local symptoms are often identical.
- **Phytotherapy.** Very important as corollary therapy to antibiotics.
- **Physical therapy.** Warm sitz baths or steam baths with addition of herbal extracts (chamomile).

15.2.4 Alternating Therapy

- **Neural therapy.** Quaddle therapy with local anesthetics over the Head's zones and associated segments.
- **Autohemotherapy.** Can be useful especially in chronic cases.

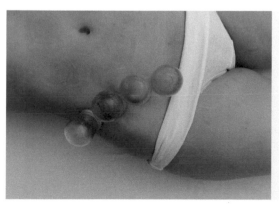

Fig. 15.2 Dry cupping along the ureter to the sacrum.

16 Nervous System

16.1 Inflammation of the Nerves (Neuritis), Neuralgia (Ischialgia)

Neuritis refers to inflammations and damage of a nerve. Its cause can be found in infectious, toxic, and mechanical vascular disorders, or in metabolic disturbances. In neuritis, the patient suffers from burning, piercing, or stabbing pain that increases at night, during movement, and with temperature changes.

Also typical for inflammations of the nerves are sensory disturbances like tingling, limbs falling asleep, and muscular weakness to the point of complete paralysis.

Neuralgia, on the other hand, refers to episodic, often excruciating pain along the course of a sensitive or mixed nerve, without any visible external changes. Neuralgic pain is wrenching or pulling, piercing or dull.

Neuralgic pain differs from the pain associated with neuritis in that it occurs in lightning-fast attacks that are often preceded by a sensation of heat or formication. The pain lasts for seconds or minutes.

Between attacks, the patient is either completely free of pain or experiences dull pain of low intensity.

> **Note**
>
> Neuritis, in contrast, manifests in permanent pain. Transition from neuritis to neuralgia is smooth.

Possible causes of neuralgia are
- Infections of all kinds.
- Metabolic disorders.
- Anemia.
- Arthritis.

Under the heading of neuralgia, we include trigeminal, intercostal, sciatic, and herpes-zoster pain, but also certain types of toothache and migraine. Many forms of unbearable neuralgic pain have a psychosomatic origin.

Ischialgia is the most common form of chronic neuralgia.

> **Note**
>
> Sciatica refers to the appearance of severe pain along the course of the sciatic nerve and its branches.

Ischialgia can be caused by injuries or pressure on the nerve, damage to the intervertebral discs, poisoning, metabolic or infectious diseases, inflammations in the area of the lower lumbar spinal column, or radiating pain from coxitis, but also quite commonly, as in lumbago, by lifting heavy objects.

16.1.1 Symptoms

- Various types of pain (stabbing, wrenching, dull), originating in the lower section of the spinal column and often running through the entire leg into the foot.
- Occasionally, numbness and weakening of the calf muscles and sensitivity in the hip. Aggravation of pain by movement, coughing, sneezing, or pressure.
- Neuralgia is difficult to affect with medication. It does, however, respond well to regulation therapies.

As in any disease, we must first consider the cause of ischialgia.

16.1.2 Suggested Therapy

Neuralgic disorders, like rheumatic ones, fall into the range of indications for cupping therapy (▶ Fig. 16.1).

Memorize	M!
Apply cupping treatment twice per week, until the complaints have disappeared.	

16.1.3 Supplemental Therapy

- **Homeopathy.** We generally prescribe the same homeopathic remedies for neuralgia and neuritis. In most cases, pain can be eliminated in a short time with organotropic and functiotropic remedies.
- **Phytotherapy.** Embrocation with external circulation-enhancing extracts increases the effect of cupping treatment.
- **Vitamins.** Vitamin B complex and vitamin E.

16.1.4 Alternating Therapy

- **Chiropractic therapy.** In *slipped disk.*
- **Neural therapy.** Quaddle therapy with local anesthetics over the corresponding segments and tender areas.
- **Acupuncture.** Causal treatment.

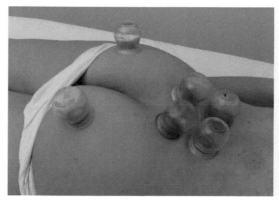

Fig. 16.1 Dry cupping on both sides of the lumbar vertebrae and above tender areas, often on the buttock cheeks and thighs. In alternating treatment, *cupping massage* brings faster results.

16.2 Disorders of the Vegetative Regulation

Whenever we speak of high blood pressure, diabetes mellitus, allergies, cancer, or back pain, we automatically think also of disorders of the vegetative regulation, which are also typical for our time.

This is how the human organism fights back against the unnatural challenges of our technological and chemical civilization. While the modern approach to nature and to humanity has made us richer in material terms and has filled our minds with great knowledge, we have not become happier or healthier. Just as we thought that scientific medicine has got all disease "under control," we realize that the highly developed civilization we have created makes us so sick that there are no fewer sick people today than in earlier times when the art of medicine only knew of few options.

As a matter of fact, because we are being flooded with unnatural stimuli and great stressors, our time is practically made to transform healthy people into chronically ill people. Constant psychological stress, constant tension from the attempt to meet challenges of today, overwhelms, especially, the vegetative nervous system, which regulates our bodily functions. Compounded by noise, environmental pollution, abuse or misuse of medications, industrially processed (devalued) foods, and interference with the natural periodicity of the human organism (e.g., chronic lack of sleep, tension without periods of relaxation), this situation leads to impaired functions and functional processes in the organism.

Because the resilience of the human organism has reached its limit, the nervous system is no longer able to regulate the necessary vital balance of all activities of the organs and organ systems. As a result, we see a frightening increase in nervous exhaustion, anxiety, cardiac and circulatory disorders, sexual dysfunctions, and chronic fatigue. Alternatively, misregulation of the unconscious (vegetative) nerves can also lead to damage in the organs and organ disease, such as heart attack, stroke, vascular disorders, stomach ulcers, etc. In addition, we can see rather less harmful but often torturous headaches, irritable bowel syndrome (IBS), back pain, painful sensations in the bones and muscles, tinnitus, dizziness, and all other vague discomforts.

Even the tender nervous system of children is taxed by ever-increasing challenges in ways that are not always suited to the organization of the young organism with regards to physical and psychological strain. As a result, such overly stressed children are often overstimulated, nervous, enraged by very minor things, show great mood swings, and complain of headaches and fatigue. Normal feelings of hunger and satiety are often impaired, which disturbs the functioning of the gastro-intestinal tract. And it is precisely these disturbances that are highly significant because they in turn impact the sustenance of the organism as a whole and reduce the ability of the weakened immune system to resist the progression of functional disturbances and from contracting other illnesses.

Note

Disturbances in the vegetative regulation can also manifest as dysregulation of individual organs or entire organ systems without measurable changes in the organ. The symptoms range from ones that are localized precisely to sensations that can change continuously in intensity and localization.

The most common disturbances are those that involve the cardiovascular system, the gastrointestinal tract, and the musculoskeletal system.

For obvious reasons, it is impossible here to describe the multiple organizations of the nervous system and the changing relationship between the individual and his or her environment in greater detail. But it is clear that the vital unconscious (vegetative) nerves, overburdened by visual or acoustic stimulation, hectic lifestyle, existential fear, family problems, or constant pressure to perform, are sounding the alarm. They are no longer able to stand up to the pressure. The result is excessive reactions that are hostile to life. As malfunctioning of the nerves provides a fertile ground for serious organic disorders, we must take note of and treat at the earliest signs of increased irritability, minor frailty, and reduced resilience in the nerves.

Vegetative organ syndromes cannot be presented as a single unit but must be described individually because of the different complaint patterns, causes, and backgrounds.

16.3 Vegetative Dystonia

Vegetative dystonia (disturbed regulation of the vegetative nervous system) refers to regulatory disturbances in individual organs or entire organ systems, without evidence of organ damage.

A relatively large number of patients who visit naturopathic practitioners suffer from vegetative dystonia.

Job- or family-related conflicts, overexertion, existential insecurity, and so on manifest as physical malfunctions. In spite of the fact that no organic changes can be noticed, patients feel very ill.

The adrenaline balance of an organism that has suffered excessive tension in this way for a long time is bound to lead to neurovegetative derailment.

16.3.1 Symptoms

The effects of these disturbances are organ-related symptoms such as
• A feeling of retching and dryness in the throat.
• Bladder irritation.
• Constipation.
• More rarely diarrhea.
• Cardiac arrhythmia.
• Pressure and stabbing pain in the heart region.
• Constricted feeling in the chest.
• Poor circulation.

The pain arises generally in the head and muscles, especially in the shoulder-neck-arm area and lower back. In addition, we see
• Sleep disturbances.
• Dizziness.
• Fear.
• Agitation.
• Fatigue and exhaustion.
• Depressive mood swings.
• Nervousness.
• Tendency to asthma and allergies.
• Sexual malfunctions.

16.3.2 Suggested Therapy

In conventional Western medicine, vegetative dystonia is mostly treated with psychotropic drugs, hypnotics, and sedatives. These remedies can provide the patient only with temporary relief. They are not truly helpful because they can additionally impede or even block vegetative regulation.

Cupping therapy, on the other hand, offers true relief. At the same time, this therapy serves to confirm or disprove the previous diagnosis of vegetative dystonia.

It is important to start specific treatment of vegetative dystonia early and not at a point when the regulatory system can no longer be activated or is already destroyed. My experiences with cupping therapy in the treatment of vegetative dystonia are so positive and convincing that I can strongly recommend this healing method. The explanation for the good treatment successes of cupping therapy in vegetative dystonia are related, among other factors, to the stimulation and mobilization of the organism's own regulatory systems.

- Treatment should begin with segmental therapy at the site of the symptoms. Repeated treatments can often suffice in segment-related disturbances to obtain a retuning of the state of vegetative reaction.
- Afterwards, treatment should be performed via the spinal column. According to acupuncture theory, one of the eight extraordinary channels, the so-called *governing vessel* (GV), which runs through the back, is in charge of regulating energy.
- In vegetative dystonia, it is also important to treat the spinal column, since this is the location where the manifold interchanges between organs and glands take place.
- Because the effect of cupping on the spinal column is stronger than on other places, you should only treat a part of the spinal column in each session (▶ Fig. 16.2, ▶ Fig. 16.3, ▶ Fig. 16.4).

The following treatment formula has proven effective—albeit with great flexibility:

Initially, **one treatment per week**, with a total of **15 treatments**. Further cupping treatments depending on effect.

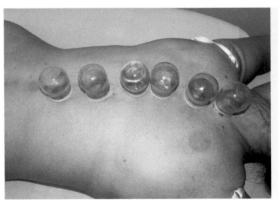

Fig. 16.2 Dry cupping above the cervical and thoracic vertebrae.

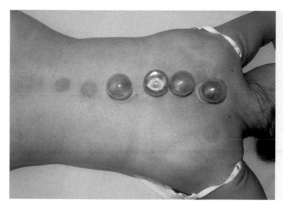

Fig. 16.3 Dry cupping above the thoracic vertebrae.

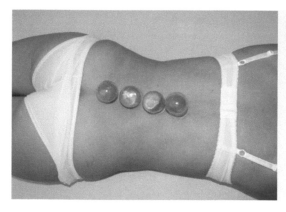

Fig. 16.4 Dry cupping above the lumbar vertebrae.

16.3.3 Supplemental Therapy

- **Homeopathy.** In this disease, the therapist encounters a person with a thousandfold complaints, from psychological behavioral disorders (like depression and fear) to organ diseases without any visible damage to the organ (such as poor digestion, bladder irritation, and angina pectoris). Most patients turn to a naturopathic practitioner because they feel ill, but nobody believes them. With personotropic homeopathic therapy, you can achieve good results.
- **Phytotherapy.** Patent medicines according to indication (St. John's wort, hawthorn, mistletoe).
- **Physical therapy.** Alternating full-body washings.

16.3.4 Alternating Therapy

Neural therapy. To achieve a retuning of the vegetative regulation, repeated intravenous injections have proven effective.

16.4 Irritable Bowel Syndrome

This syndrome is one of the most common disorders seen in general medical practice. It belongs to a group of vegetative regulation disorders that are also referred to as psychosomatic disorders. Initially, no organ damage is detectable in the individual organs, but considerable disturbances are present nevertheless.

Nevertheless, IBS is in no way a purely psychosomatic disorder. In most cases, this disorder has a long history, and the excessive sensitivity of the nervous system in the gastrointestinal tract has existed for a long time already (e.g., after infectious bowel disease, allergic conditions in earlier years, but also toxic influences, side effects of medications, fasting diet). This allows psychological stress and tension (e.g., chronic worrying, emergencies, grief, constant stress) to trigger or increase a functional disturbance in the bowel.

As a result, the psychological stress and tension cause an increased flow of nerve impulses from the brain, which reach the muscles of the intestinal walls via the nervous system. As the central organ of the nervous system, the brain, is intimately connected via the individual nerve tracts to the nerves of the digestive system. Consequently, the activities that take place in the brain also radiate outward to a greater or lesser extent into the organs of the gastrointestinal tract. Disturbances in the digestive function with associated symptoms are a result of this connection.

As IBS causes many and varied complaints, the patient may be suspected of suffering from a malign bowel disease or intestinal cancer. However, contradicting this, in most cases, is the fact that the patient is in good general health in spite of the often chronic complaints. Nevertheless, the diagnosis of IBS can only be given after the possibility of real organ disease has been eliminated, even if you suspect IBS. It is, after all, possible that other disorders are present, e.g.:

- Lactose intolerance.
- Celiac disease.
- Thyroid dysfunction.
- Intestinal infection.
- Inflammatory bowel disease.
- Crohn's disease.
- Diverticulitis.
- Ulcerative colitis.
- Intestinal cancer.

After the physical diagnosis has confirmed no organically identifiable causes, the complaints should not be devalued or trivialized. An "irritable bowel" is, after all, not an imagined disease but a neural dysfunction in the abdominal area that constantly causes these symptoms and therefore makes the patient's social and professional life miserable.

Lastly, we should note at this point that the transition to the organic processes is fluid and that the chronic functional disturbances can certainly contribute to an earlier occurrence of pathological changes in the bowel. This will, in turn, lead to the development of disturbances in the resorption or the metabolic processes, and manifest as other disorders.

16.4.1 Symptoms

- The most common symptom is intestinal spasms that are caused by excessive cramping in the muscles of the intestinal walls.

- Diarrhea and constant strong bloating and constipation can occur alternatingly. Sometimes we also see mucous in the stool.
- In addition, there can be gastric discomfort, a feeling of fullness, increased intestinal sounds (rumbling, borborygmus), burning and pressing abdominal pain, frequent belching, and increased flatulence.
- In some cases, we can see intolerance to the consumption of certain foods, nausea, heartburn, difficulty in swallowing, lack of appetite, and internal agitation.
- It is typical for complaints to occur right after waking and to increase throughout the course of the day. Complaints at night are exceptions.
- The complaints themselves can in turn lead to psychological problems. Thus, it is not rare that anxiety, nervousness, depression, and increased sensitivity to noises, smells, light, cold, or warmth might develop.
- Normally, extra-abdominal symptoms exist concomitantly, such as disturbed circulatory regulation, tachycardia, paresthesia in the heart, Roemheld syndrome, tension-related back and joint pain, frequent urination, vasomotor headaches, and menstrual complaints.

16.4.2 Suggested Therapy

It is obvious that in such cases a therapy that is only oriented toward the symptoms, such as prescribing pain killers, laxatives, antidiarrheals, or antacids, which will only achieve temporary results, will not be effective. Irritable bowel syndrome requires a therapy that is suitable for eliminating the hypersensitivity of the gastrointestinal tract to the point where the stimuli are no longer able to trigger the neural malfunctions in the abdominal area. At the same time, therapy should restore normal intestinal functions.

> **Note**
>
> For this reason, treatment consists of a meaningful combination of cupping, homeopathy, phytotherapy, and general measures. Of course, it is not always necessary to maximize treatment. We should always consider which elements are individually suited to each patient. In this context, it has proven very effective to take a complex approach to IBS.

Treatment results are good but often not long-lasting. Because the tolerance level for certain stimuli has been lowered for a long time, it makes sense that it cannot be raised quickly but often remains stubbornly persistent even when the complaints are reduced or improved. For this reason, not only long-term therapy but also patience and perseverance in the interaction with the patient are required.

Cupping presents an excellent foundational therapy that can raise the lowered sensitivity threshold back up through a readjustment and reduce the hypersensitivity of the gastrointestinal tract. For this purpose, the cups are applied to certain reflex zones or to the appropriate acupuncture points (▶ Fig. 16.5, ▶ Fig. 16.6, ▶ Fig. 16.7, ▶ Fig. 16.8).

As already mentioned, it is necessary to perform a flexible treatment that is completely attuned to the patient. In this context, the following treatment schedule has proven effective: Initially **1 treatment per week with a cupping duration of 4 minutes.** If you proceed with caution, there is no need to fear of uncomfortable reactions.

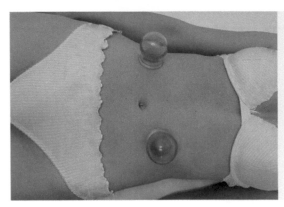

Fig. 16.5 Below the ribs: Disturbances of the digestive tract such as bloating.

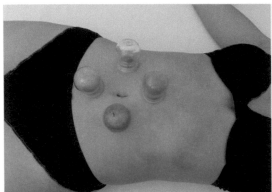

Fig. 16.6 On the abdomen: Lack of responsiveness.

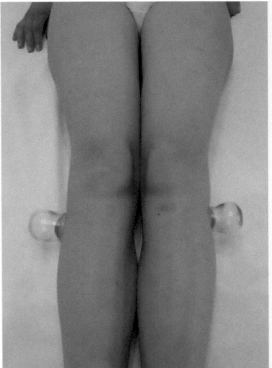

Fig. 16.7 On the legs: Fears and nervousness—harmonization points.

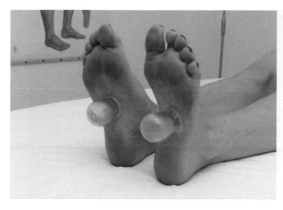

Fig. 16.8 On the foot reflex zones of the digestive tract alternating with the foot reflex zone solar plexus, as in ▶ Fig. 16.11.

Subsequently, you can consider a more frequent treatment, **twice per week, with a cupping duration of 10 minutes.** After a clear improvement has been achieved, treatment intervals should initially be **14 days**. Later on, the chronic nature of the condition may require continued treatment **once per month** for an extended period of time.

If it becomes apparent that a relapse threatens, intervals should temporarily be shortened again.

If pain is felt during cupping on the foot reflex zones, please note the warning in chapter 3.3.

16.4.3 Supplemental Therapy

Homeopathy

In IBS, homeopathy offers a good treatment option. This fact becomes more significant when we recall that this disorder is among the more common ones. Because of the variability of symptoms, the choice of remedy is quite difficult. As such, this disorder first raises the question how many remedies we should prescribe at the same time or in alternation. Experience shows that a single remedy, such as was done in Hahnemann's times, is not sufficient. While it is often only a single remedy that leads to healing, it is equally true that some disorders require several remedies simultaneously or alternatingly, in order to achieve good treatment results.

Dr. Samuel Hahnemann was able to achieve astounding results with single remedies, but more than 200 years have passed since then. During this time period, significant changes have occurred in the state of the environment, in diseases, and in the reactions of the organism in health and in illness. The proven classical treatment with a single remedy, of course, continues to be predominant, but it is clear in contemporary clinical practice that an accurately chosen remedy must still be supplemented by one or more others.

Phytotherapy

The use of different plant-based substances that are appropriate for the needs of the patient is recommended. It is impossible to predict which plants are effective in an individual case. Tried and tested plants are: fennel, gypsyweed, chamomile, peppermint leaf, sage, caraway, lemonbalm, hawthorn flowers, calamus (sweet flag) root, angelica.

Pulverized flaxseeds have a normalizing effect in cases of both constipation and diarrhea. They have also proven effective for hyperacidity, gastritis, fermentative dyspepsia, and to inhibit the growth of putrefying bacteria in the intestines.

General Measures

It is important to explain the connections between the various symptoms to the patient. Because of complaints like intestinal spasm, bloating, borborygmus, and persistent constipation or diarrhea, many patients understandably develop fears that a malign tumor may be present. It is our job to allay the patient's fear of a malign disease. In general, though, a mere understanding of the connections is not enough. The process of "letting go" of deep fears is not easy and takes place over an extended period of time.

Memorize	M!
Compassionate guidance gives the patient a chance to get a grip on his or her disorder through a meaningful therapy. It is important to emphasize repeatedly that this requires patience and that the possibility of relapses must be taken into account in the beginning.	

In this context, psychotherapy can be helpful and useful, as long as it is not utilized as the only therapy. Physical treatment is often the right therapy choice, and in some cases psychotherapy is not indicated.

Patients who cannot be helped in overcoming their fear through talking can often make good progress with the help of hypnosis.

We should also assess which method is most appropriate for the individual patient. It is important to avoid psychological situations that make the patient ill as much as possible.

Because patients often comment that the complaints are amplified by prolonged sitting in front of the computer or at a desk or after long trips in the car, consistent physical activity is important.

Dietetics

A strict dietary program is not necessary. Foods that cause bloating and promote fermentation in the intestines should be avoided. It seems useful to split the usual amount of food into smaller meals to be taken throughout the day and to always consume the meal without rushing.

Some patients may need supplementary vitamins or minerals or digestive enzymes.

16.5 Burn-out Syndrome

Memorize	M!
The term burn-out refers to a certain abnormal state of the nervous system that is marked by complete physical, mental, and emotional exhaustion.	

The causes for this psycho-physiological syndrome of overextension, which has become increasingly common in the last 40 years, are varied. It is often the case that work-related, societal, and personal factors come together. Special risk factors are constant pressure to perform in one's job as well as increasing general economic insecurity and related stress and existential fears. The struggle for survival, which is more tenacious and invasive in the present times than in previous centuries, places the nervous system into a state of red alert. The activity of the nerves is kept in constant tension. This tension triggers different additional reactions. Increased amounts of stress hormones, adrenaline, and others are released into the blood; this may lead to disturbed experiences, functions, and organ reactions.

There are no detectable organic findings.

To a certain extent, stress reactions and demanding challenges are normal. On the other hand, though, it is easy to imagine that persistent rushing, pressure, negative stress, or fear of potential threats and the resulting constant psychological tension can quickly exhaust the strength of the nerves.

Unfortunately, many employers who strive for "always more" have not yet recognized this problem and demand that the high demands that they place on their employees are more than just fulfilled. The workflow and procedures that are no longer fully comprehensible today force people into a vehement time pressure. This negative sickening stress at work is then often brought back home and deprives people of the ability to relax and sleep. As a result, an increasing tension builds up that eventually can no longer be released even during vacations. In spite of this, work continues with ever more engagement. The daily routine falls by the wayside, personal needs are repressed, hobbies and family neglected. In this way, the person loses the balance between what is possible and what is necessary. As a consequence, we see a continuous aggravation of functional physical complaints and psychological disorders, which at some point leads to complete physical and mental collapse.

In this context, we can quote the words of the German journalist and author J. Freudenreich: "To work oneself to death is the only socially acceptable form of suicide."

The affected person can overlook these complaints and live for a long time with these overload risk factors. And when functional physical complaints and psychological disorders do arise, the state of exhaustion, weakness, and irritation of the nervous system is already far advanced.

Burn-out syndrome is thus a condition that develops latently after long-term overstraining and permanent tension, especially when the natural rhythm between activity —both physical and mental—and relaxation is ignored. The lack of relaxation and recuperation deprives the organism of the possibility to regenerate, and it is weakened progressively to the point where it can only offer weak resistance to the progressing disease. Sooner or later, such a person is physically and mentally exhausted, apathetic, or in other words "burned out."

The immune deficiency and frequent infections that make the life of such a person even more difficult also affect the weakened organism.

If we can recognize the earliest warning signals of the body, soul, and spirit (such as more frequent nervous irritation, disturbed sleep, heart palpitations, mental fatigue), we can generally prevent the onset of burn-out syndrome by means of a holistic therapy. Understandably, it is more cost efficient and sensible to implement preventative measures than to have the patient undergo a long, expensive, and intensive medical treatment of a fully developed disease.

16.5.1 Symptoms

The effects of an overburdened nervous system become apparent both in physical as well as mental manifestations. Typical symptoms are:
• Mood swings.
• Irritability.
• Lack of motivation.
• Chronic fatigue.
• Internal restlessness.
• Reduced ability to relax, sleep disturbances.
• Anxiety.
• Excessive sweating.
• Lack of appetite.
• Depression, resignation, apathy.
• Often at the same time hyperactivity.
• Often a feeling of stiffness arises all over the body along with muscle tension (painful, knotty hardenings, so-called myogelosis) and hence tension-related shoulder, neck, or back pain or headaches can occur.
• It is also common to see the circulation and gastrointestinal tract affected. This can lead to symptoms or complaints triggered by warmth, cold, or weather, or to sexual dysfunctions.
• Because of the permanent stress, the immune system is irritated and weakened, and this immune deficiency can result in frequent infections.

16.5.2 Suggested Therapy

Fortunately, natural medicine also has methods for this condition at its disposal, to prevent the person's health from worsening. A combined treatment of cupping, homeopathy, phytotherapy, and lifestyle adjustments aims to substantially improve the general state of health in a short time, within a few weeks, and thereby to steer the patient away from a full outbreak of the pathological pattern. Nevertheless, the treatment must be continued over a longer period of time to avoid a relapse, even after therapeutic effects have become visible.

It is almost impossible to avoid stress nowadays. As such, any measures that calm the psyche and release tension and that are able to correct the problems with the regulatory capacity of the organism are highly recommended. Because cupping has a soothing, relaxing, and mood-changing effect, it can offer a valuable contribution in this context. The patient's physical and psychological equilibrium are restored and strengthened.

A treatment schedule can only be given with caveats since a flexible approach is a must. The following schedule has proven effective:

Initially, carry out **2 treatments per week.** There are two different paths to choose from for the treatment: In the first session, apply the cups along the spinal column (▶ Fig. 16.9); in the second session, apply them to the feet (solar plexus zones; ▶ Fig. 16.11) and legs. Alternatively: In the first session, put the cups next to the shoulder blades (▶ Fig. 16.10) and on the feet (solar plexus zones); in the second session, put them next to the shoulder blades and on the legs.

Following this, treatment should take place **every 3 weeks.** This therapy is continued until you can be sure that the goal is achieved.

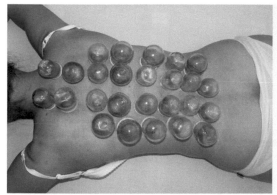

Fig. 16.9 Dry cupping on both sides of the spinal column.

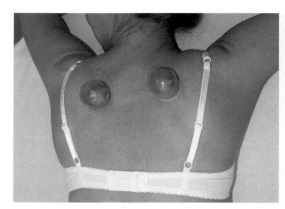

Fig. 16.10 Dry cupping next to the shoulder blades: Exhaustion, weakness, anxiety, neurasthenia, convalescence.

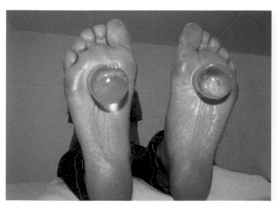

Fig. 16.11 Dry cupping on the foot reflex zones solar plexus.

Note

Dry cupping on the legs as in ▶ Fig. 16.7.

16.5.3 Supplemental Therapy

Homeopathy

When remedies are used with patience, burn-out syndrome can be prevented, if psychotropic drugs or other stronger chemical remedies are not preferred.

There is a large choice of remedies available that can be used for burn-out syndrome. Because of the diversity of symptoms, however, the selection can be difficult. For psychological and physical complaints that have been present for weeks already, the use of several remedies at the same time or alternatingly has proven effective, in order to get results as quickly as possible. This is admittedly a stopgap solution, but it is often impossible to draw conclusions from the diffused syndrome for a single effective remedy. You could use each remedy for a week, but will lose a lot of time in the process.

The question always arises whether you should prescribe several homeopathic remedies simultaneously. Many homeopaths have a skeptical, if not completely disapproving, attitude toward prescribing several remedies at the same time. In essence, this rejection is based in the homeopathic perspective.

The term homeopathy only refers to the form of treatment known to be in accordance with Dr. Samuel Hahnemann's rules. We call it "classical homeopathy" for a compelling reason: It has many descendants today that strictly speaking do not conform to these rules but whose value is undeniable. Ever since many practitioners have recognized that the prescription of several remedies simultaneously is able to greatly influence even conditions that are difficult to affect, homeopathic remedies have become increasingly important. Additionally, it is a part of the job of a practitioner to vary treatment from one patient to another. For this reason, many practitioners turn to the less classical path of homeopathy, if it means that they are able to help their patients without forcefully suppressing symptoms by means of chemical preparations that can even cause addiction.

Phytotherapy

The following herbs that can be combined according to the needs of the individual patient are recommended: *Lemonbalm, hawthorn fruits and leaves, hops, St. John's wort, rosemary, peppermint, mistletoe*, and *lavender*.

Beneficial effect can be achieved with alcohol-based extracts of *valerian root, motherwort*, and *oat*.

General Measures

A key requirement in the treatment of burn-out syndrome, which is, however, difficult to fulfill, is the removal of the causes that lead to the overextension of the nervous system in the first place. For this reason, it is important to aspire to a natural life rhythm and to pay attention to a regular daily routine. Any chance of causing tension, excitement, or overstimulation in the nerves should be carefully avoided. Leisure time should be exclusively for relaxation and recuperation. Sufficient sleep is essential. Any kind of physical and mental work should only be performed to the appropriate degree so that you can restore the strength of the nervous system. Activities in fresh air, like bicycling, hiking, and working in the garden are important. For many patients, spending time in a beautiful natural environment (free of external stimuli) is recommended.

The soul and the spirit as well as the body need sufficient strengthening, but without excessive strain.

Dietetics

No special diet but simple food, as natural as possible and balanced, should be eaten because radical changes to one's former eating habits frequently lead to tension, which stands in the way of healing.

17 Venous Disorders

17.1 Varicose Veins (Varices)

Varicose veins are found in approximately 35% of all adults. The degree of pathology varies substantially depending on the extent, type, and location.

Primary varices develop in predisposed individuals on the basis of congenital weakness of the vein walls. *Secondary varices* are most commonly the result of past thrombophlebitis.

Nevertheless, degenerative processes in the vein walls can also play a role, as adaptation to constant false or excessive strain after blockages.

Varicose veins can also develop from prolonged standing, pinching clothing, chronic constipation or obesity.

Finally, pregnancy also frequently leads to cardiac edemas and varices.

17.1.1 Symptoms

- Tingling, feeling of coldness or heaviness, and pain in the legs, especially after prolonged sitting or standing.
- Feet and joints can swell.
- Nightly cramps in the calf.

17.1.2 Suggested Therapy

The treatment of varicose veins is one of the main applications of cupping, increasing blood circulation and accelerating the discharge of infectious fluid collections. By cupping, you can decongest the area of the damaged vessel and prevent the formation of varicose veins.

The following therapy protocol has proven to be reliable: Dry cupping in the crease between the buttocks and thighs. **Initially three to four treatments per week.** Depending on success, repeat treatments **every 5 or 7 days.**

> **Note**
>
> Before a patient decides to undergo surgery to remove varicose veins, it is worth applying cupping therapy, which can often avoid surgical intervention. Although the patient may experience relief after surgery, the old state often returns within only a few years.

> **Memorize** M!
>
> In pronounced varicosis, the two methods of varicosclerozation and stripping cannot be used. In such cases, only consistent treatment with cupping and compression is effective.

17.1.3 Supplemental Therapy

- Elevate legs during rest and apply wraps and compressive bandages or **compression stockings**, which should be worn continuously, especially in cases with leg edema.
- **Regulate bowel movements**.
- **Physical therapy:** Physical measures and active vascular training are of great significance. Foot baths including the calf with the addition of chestnut, walnut leaf, oak bark, witch-hazel, or rosemary extract, water temperature ca. 30°C (86°F), **length of bath 10 minutes.** Daily cold affusions (lower and upper leg) increase the pumping capacity of the calf muscles.

> ### Caution! ⚠
>
> - In acute inflammations, do not apply hydrotherapy or balneotherapy!
> - Caution in massage! The areas around varicose veins must not be massaged.
> - When applying herbal extracts, ointments, and compresses that have a circulation-stimulating effect, beware that the irritated skin does not tolerate every ointment and often also does not tolerate herbal extracts or compresses that irritate the skin.

- **Phytotherapy.** The combination of plant-based medicines and cupping has proven effective. Chestnut preparations increase the velocity of the blood flow and venous backflow. They have a tonifying effect on arteries and veins. *Witch-hazel* is a popular remedy in venous disorders, applied both internally and externally.
- **Homeopathy.** Homeopathy is a good choice for treating disorders of the venous system. Select remedies in accordance with individual symptoms and use for longer periods.

18 Obesity (Adipositas, Overweight)

18.1 General Remarks

It is not without special reason that I have added obesity to this book, because not everybody is aware that cupping is very useful in the reduction of excess weight. The patient is able to observe convincing results quickly, gain trust in the treatment of obesity with cupping, and hence be motivated to persevere in losing weight.

Obesity is not a disease in itself but a symptom. Nevertheless, this state means that the entire organism is overburdened, as a result of which the risk factors for other diseases frequently arise in obese patients.

With rare exceptions (disease of the internal glands), the primary cause of obesity is found in a long-term disturbance of the ratio between energy intake and consumption, facilitated by the intake of too many calories with a diet that is too rich and a lack of physical exercise.

The correct functioning of the metabolism is of prime importance in overweight patients.

Losing weight is difficult for most obese people. Many have tried the various available diets and have occasionally achieved considerable weight loss with drastic starvation diets, only to lapse back into obesity after a short time. Unfortunately, the weight loss of several pounds occurring so promisingly in the first week of a starvation diet is only an illusion. The reason for this is that this loss rests largely on a removal of water, not fat. Fasting diets and diuretic drugs bring only temporary success because the body usually reestablishes its water balance quite quickly. These diets are therefore often frustrating.

While currently available appetite inhibitors do make losing weight easier, they are not tenable over time. In most cases, such remedies are not completely without risks.

In the treatment of obesity, we therefore have to prioritize the following measures. With the exception of a few cases of obesity caused by endocrine factors, its treatment consists primarily of
- Correcting lifestyle and eating habits.
- Creating an appropriate dietary plan.
- Stimulation of the metabolism.

Effectively reducing weight requires a lot of patience and psychological readjustment. Patience is necessary because these are all measures that must be performed over many months. It is of little benefit to a person's health to lose something like 15 kg in a short period of time. Neither can most people afford the time or energy to undergo an austere fast or diet for so many weeks or months that it prevents them from fulfilling their professional obligations and experiencing a normal life.

We must take into consideration that modern humans have mostly lost their healthy instincts. With regard to nutrition, this manifests in a lack of moderation in the intake of food. People continue to eat long after their hunger has been satisfied. Simple lack of movement aggravates this situation further.

Limiting calorie intake can only be achieved by eating less and with a heightened awareness of calories. This requires a psychological readjustment. Permanent weight loss cannot be achieved by dieting alone. Real treatment of obesity remains incomplete without a fundamental correction of lifestyle and eating habits.

Because the feeling of satiation depends primarily on the amount of consumed food in most obese patients, the change in eating habits should focus less on limiting the amount than on making the proper selection of foods. For example, a low-fat diet, if followed consistently, achieves reliable results. With a proper selection of foods, an overweight person can eat until satiated without ingesting large amounts of calories. Additional calories can be saved with a glass of mineral water or a yogurt before meals because these fill the stomach and reduce hunger as well as the amount of consumed foods.

In this way, overweight people can gradually lose weight over the course of months or even years.

At the same time, however, an increase in physical exercise has to occur consistently and permanently, to achieve a higher energy consumption.

Healthy metabolic performance and a well-functioning endocrine system determine whether a person is obese or thin with equal food intake. If these positive preconditions are missing, **cupping treatment** revitalizes metabolic processes and stimulates endocrine functions.

In this context, we take advantage of the experience of cupping as a regulation therapy. Here, the metabolic processes are not influenced by means of artificial drugs, but the weakened endocrine function is retuned and stimulated.

Healthy and vital cellular functioning also includes the elimination of excess water from the tissue, an important prerequisite for the loss of excess weight. As a result of cupping, the stimulated circulation increases the velocity of the blood flow, which in turn leads to a faster discharge of excess water from the tissue. In addition, cupping strengthens peristalsis and thereby regulates bowel movements, which can further be supported by appropriate diet and exercise. Cupping therapy not only serves as an important supportive measure, but also helps in maintaining the elasticity of the skin while losing weight.

18.2 Suggested Therapy

The art of losing weight hinges on never letting the patient experience a feeling of hunger because most overweight people, after many diets, are afraid of hunger.

The following therapy protocol has proven to be reliable: **Dry cupping** on the abdomen, in the lumbar region, in the crease between the thigh and buttock. As **basic regulation,** treatment initially occurs **two to three times per week,** with a **course of treatment lasting 4–6 weeks.** Afterwards, treatment occurs **once a week over 6 weeks.** Following this, **one treatment every 2 weeks** for a long period of time, to maintain the effect.

Continuing treatment is extremely important for maintaining the achieved stimulation of the regulatory cycle and for allowing the therapist to supervise continuously and direct the progress in losing weight.

18.3 Supplemental Therapy

- **Homeopathy.** The use of appropriate homeopathic remedies can strengthen the stimulation of the fat metabolism.
- **Treatment with medication** is only necessary when concomitant diseases exist.

19 Cellulitis (Adipositas Circumscripta Oedematosa); Cellulite (Dermopanniculosis Deformans)

19.1 General Remarks

In spite of the fact that cellulitis is not considered a serious medical problem, it can have a psychological effect. Even well-proportioned young women with slim legs can have colossal thighs. The external appearance of the skin surface is reinforced by domed irregularities. In a society in which a perfect body is an expression of beauty, youth, and productivity, cellulitis has become a source of great fear for many women, who are disproportionately affected by this disorder (approximately 90%). Among men, only 3% suffer from cellulitis.

With the hormonal changes related to puberty, girls form more fat and thereby assume their typical female shape—broader hips, a round bottom, a slender waist, and plump breasts. Adolescent boys, in contrast, develop more muscle mass. Both connective tissue and skin are structured differently and are clearly weaker in women than in men. The female fat cells that are stored in the subcutaneous tissue are larger and positioned more densely under the skin than the male cells. In a slim woman with normal weight, roughly a quarter of this can be fat, while it is only 12–14% of a man's normal weight. These differences in body structure explain why cellulitis is primarily a problem in women and why the storage of fat cells not necessarily means overweight.

Cellulitis is defined as circumscribed fat storage (adipositas circumscripta oedematosa) with mild lymph congestion and edema formation in the area of the connective tissue, especially on women's thighs. **Cellulite** (dermopanniculosis deformans) refers to changes in the structure of the subcutaneous tissue, especially changes in the connective tissue, which separates the individual fat lobes from each other. The fat cell chambers can thereby become deformed, as a result of which the skin area appears quilted, initially only when pinched and later spontaneously. We speak of "orange peel" or "mattress" skin.

Two types of fat storage exist. In one, the number of fat cells increases, which leads to obesity due to cellular reproduction. In the other, the stored fat cells themselves increase in size.

Because the chronic pressure of enlarged fat cells inhibits the flow of blood and lymph, it disturbs the local metabolism that continuously takes place in every cell and in the bodily fluids. Little by little, this reduces nutrients as well as oxygen. At the same time, it inhibits the removal of metabolic waste products. As a result of this chronic nutritional deficiency and accumulation of metabolic waste products, the texture of the smallest blood vessels, as well as of the connective tissue in which the fat lobes are embedded, changes. As a result, we see palpable hardened knots, and, due to the congestion of lymph, the formation of edemas.

The fat reserves and tissue changes can only be prevented if the metabolism functions correctly. A normal metabolism is, after all, a prerequisite for the trouble-free execution of nutritional and detoxifying functions in all parts of the organism.

19.2 Suggested Therapy

Not starvation diets, but a nutritional program that pursues the goal of balancing out misdirected metabolic processes with an optimal composition. The main reason why cellulitis successfully resists dieting attempts is well known. Most diets are extremely low in calories. The body's protective mechanisms respond to a diet that demands a drastic reduction in calories not only with increased hunger signals but also by adjusting the basic requirements and speed of metabolism. The body does not see a difference between a voluntary reduction of calories and involuntary starvation, as can happen during famines. In both cases, the body slows down its metabolism to preserve as much energy as possible.

For the treatment of cellulitis, cupping massage is recommended. Nevertheless, cupping massage can initially be quite painful on the affected locations and can therefore be quickly abandoned by many women.

> **Memorize** **M!**
>
> Because the thighs are the most painful locations for both cupping and cupping massage, we recommend using small suction cups and a weak suction force for the first treatment. A lesser suction force can also be obtained by a small flame.

In the first session, the application should last **no longer than 5 minutes.** Further treatments are determined by the patient's tolerance to cupping or cupping massage and by treatment success.

Treatment can be supported by sufficient fluid intake as well as exercise such as bicycling or swimming.

19.3 Supplemental Therapy

- **Phytotherapy.** Tea infusions or patent medicines that promote the metabolism and the elimination of excess water from the tissue.
- **Homeopathy.** A homeopathic course of treatment for liver, kidneys, and intestine is recommended. The remedies must be selected on an individual basis.

20 Weather Sensitivity and Weather-Triggered Symptoms and Complaints

20.1 Note

Whoever knows the origin of the winds, the thunder, and the weather also knows where illness comes from.

Paracelsus

Disease progression and the state of health can be affected not just from the inside, but also from the outside, through a variety of factors. Especially, the weather triggers health-related changes in some people, both in a negative and positive sense.

It has been known for centuries that many people react to certain meteorological parameters with a decline in well-being. Aristotle (384–322 BCE), Hippocrates (460–377 BCE), Paracelsus (1493–1541), Alexander von Humboldt (1796–1859), and others observed that the weather can change the physical, mental, and emotional state of a person.

Regarding the biological effect of the weather on humans, we can distinguish three different responses:
- Normal reaction.
- Weather sensitivity.
- Weather-triggered symptom or complaint.

When meteorological parameters, such as atmospheric pressure, temperature, light conditions, or humidity, change greatly and quickly and trigger immediate physical and/or psychological complaints in a person, this is called **weather sensitivity.** In contrast, when a change in weather has an activating or aggravating effect on the complaints and symptoms of already existing illnesses in a person, we refer to this as a **weather-triggered symptom or complaint.**

As such, the terms weather sensitivity and weather-triggered refer to a reaction of the weakened organism to the change in weather, which can negatively impact the person's general state of health, mood, and productivity.

We can view the connection between the weather and the human organism from this perspective: Whether heat or cold, rain or sunshine, the organism is continuously adapting to changes in temperature and atmospheric pressure. In addition, light conditions, air movements, and humidity all require an adaptive response from the organism as well. Not every person, however, senses this process consciously since the human body is designed to create an internal milieu that is as stable as possible in spite of the changes in the external environment. The nervous system thus processes the stimuli received by the organism (environmental influences) without the person noticing it. It is only when the nervous system is overextended and unable to adapt quickly enough to the new atmospheric environmental conditions that disturbed functions and reactions in the organism might result.

Generally speaking, changes in the weather do not cause illness, but fluctuations do mean a greater strain on the autonomous regulatory systems of the organism. Rapid weather changes in particular are a strong stimulus for the organism because they require a rapid adaptation. If a person is already suffering from a weakened capacity for self-regulation due to mental, emotional, or physical strain or tension, even mild meteorological factors are able to attack the weak points in the organism, which can lead to bad reactions and to the occurrence of corresponding complaints (symptoms).

Thus, a lowered personal stimulus threshold is always a prerequisite. For this reason, some people respond more sensitively to a change in weather than others.

In order for the organism to maintain its complicated operation and thereby its health, productivity, and well-being, undisturbed adaptive processes are necessary. Nevertheless, the massive increase in environmental pollution and the manifold effects of our modern civilization present unnatural challenges for the organism that often overtax its adaptability. As a result, we see an ever increasing number of patients presenting with these complaints in today's clinical practices.

Therapy can rectify these difficulties in the organism's ability to adapt. The use of biological therapies is, therefore, more necessary today than ever before.

First, you should clarify the complaints (symptoms) described by the patient so that you can either preclude an organic cause or confirm another cause (existing illness) whose symptoms are aggravated by the weather change in spite of the best possible medicinal therapy.

20.2 Symptoms

- Complaints vary from case to case. We can see disturbances in normal physiological functions that manifest in the cardiovascular system, such as fluctuations in blood pressure or in circulation.
- Some people respond with disturbed concentration, increased irritability, disturbed sleep, depressed moods, digestive problems, headaches, or fatigue.
- Very often, we see an intensification of the symptoms that can be associated with a certain basic illness (e.g., bronchial asthma, angina pectoris, chronic polyarthritis, migraines, etc.)
- Not uncommon is sensitivity to pain in scars and injuries.
- Nevertheless, the weather also has beneficial effects on health and can contribute to an alleviation of existing complaints.

20.3 Suggested Therapy

We have to take the weather as it is, but cupping, homeopathy, phytotherapy, and general measures can help to mitigate or eliminate complaints that arise from a change in weather. In addition, treatment can also help to reduce sensitivity to weather changes to the point where the organism is able to adapt more quickly to them in the future.

For **treatment with cups** (dry cupping), the following treatment schedule has proven effective: Initially, **2 treatments per week, for a total of 12 treatments,** hence a treatment length of **4–6 weeks**. Following this, a treatment session every **3–4 weeks** for an extended period of time. Continuing treatment is important so that the achieved improvement can be maintained.

> **Note**
>
> On the first day of treatment, dry cupping on both sides along the spinal column (see ▶ Fig. 13.7).
> For the second treatment, dry cupping on top of the spinal column (see ▶ Fig. 16.2).
> As additional treatment, dry cupping on the foot reflex zone solar plexus (see ▶ Fig. 16.11).

20.3.1 Homeopathy

Homeopathy offers multiple treatment options for patients with weather sensitivity.

Individually tailored and correctly chosen remedies (i.e., in accordance with symptoms, modalities, constitution, etc.) are able to alleviate complaints and strengthen the organism against irritation from weather changes. The nervous system is supported, so that the adaptive processes are able to respond to any change in the weather in due time.

20.3.2 Phytotherapy

Particularly well suited to supporting the vegetative nervous system are herbal teas made out of *lemon balm, lavender flower, willow bark, licorice root, peppermint*, and *cistus (rock rose)*.

20.3.3 General Measures

For patients with weather sensitivity or intolerance, it is important that they go for a long walk daily, if possible, in every kind of weather (of course, except for storms and thunderstorms), to induce the adaptation of the nervous system to weather changes. Sauna sessions or alternating hot and cold baths/showers also help the body to come to terms with the constantly changing meteorological parameters in the environment. If the organism is weakened from existing illnesses, it is recommended to harden the body carefully.

In this context, sufficient sleep and good relaxation, both physical and mental, are of particular importance.

20.3.4 Dietetics

It is good to avoid heavy large meals; smaller meals throughout the day are preferable.

21 Cupping as Supportive Therapy within Conventional Western Medicine

21.1 Integrating Conventional Western Medicine and Naturopathic Healing Methods—A Possibility?

One person may proceed by anatomical examination of morbidities, another by clinical observation of processes, the third by pathological and the fourth by therapeutic experimentation, one by chemical or physical and yet another by historical research. Yet science is large enough to encompass all these directions as long as they do not want to be exclusive, overstep their boundaries, or pretend to achieve everything. Exaggerated promises have always done harm, exaggerated claims have always caused injuries, and self-aggrandizement has always offended others or ridiculed itself.

Rudolf Virchow

The intention of this chapter is to encourage representatives of clinical medicine to apply cupping without prejudice, if it leads to recovery from or even only improvement of diseases or complaints.

For this purpose, I first want to give a short summary of my own thoughts and experiences, also taking into consideration the experiences of other authors from ancient and modern times.

The issue of compatibility between conventional Western and naturopathic medicine is raised again and again in modern science because the reasoning of scientific medicine, molded as it is by chemistry and technology, differs substantially from the thinking of experiential medicine.

This is, however, very surprising since experiential medicine is the original source of science-based conventional medicine.

> **Note**
>
> The goal of any therapy is the complete restoration of health.

In this light, it should be fundamentally irrelevant whether this goal is achieved by means of conventional or naturopathic medicine.

Nevertheless, people argue over and over about which therapeutic method is more correct, "true," or truly rational.

Conventional medicine is frequently based on the premise that only those treatment methods are correct whose efficacy can be proven with technical measuring tools or statistics. Since the way in which a large variety of therapies function cannot be proven or measured directly, these are often dismissed as belonging to "outsider medicine" and their effect is referred to as placebo or superstition.

In this way, many valuable naturopathic methods continue to be rejected or derided to this day because they supposedly stem from "lay circles."

It is hereby forgotten, though, that all widely known measures recognized by conventional medicine, such as *massage* and *dietary* or *physical* treatment methods, have their origin not in the universities, but in experience and in the popularly transmitted art of healing. In our times, they have merely been refined and put on strict medical foundations. They now serve as proven treatment methods to supplement modern medicine effectively and sensibly and can even replace it in many cases.

Naturopathic medicine almost exclusively utilizes therapeutic principles that were by no means unknown in conventional Western medicine but, for whatever reasons, have been abandoned.

It is only after therapies of conventional Western medicine fail to bring a cure or improvement that naturopathic measures are occasionally permitted.

A certain amount of reservation against dubious therapeutic methods and those that transcend its possibilities and limitations is an understandable, even necessary means of protection against excessive promises, which, in most cases, harm the patient seeking help.

A wholesale rejection of naturopathic treatment methods, on the other hand, is unreasonable, unfounded, and most often rooted in an emotional aversion, in prejudices, or in a lack of knowledge and willingness to familiarize oneself properly with the other side of medicine.

How else could anyone say "I think nothing of naturopathic methods" without ever having tried them!

Naturopathic medicine can often deliver surprising results that cannot be explained in exact scientific terms. We should accept this and let the rules apply.

As we know, the human body is composed of individual parts like the trunk, extremities, head, organs, organ systems, and so on, but the holistic activity of body parts and systems only occurs on the basis of continuous, mutually dependent interrelationships underneath the connecting unity of the nervous system. No part of the human body, no organ or organ system functions on its own.

21.2 How are the Terms "Disease" and "Health" Defined within Both of These Disciplines?

Conventional medicine defines **"disease"** as "An interruption, cessation, or disorder of body functions, systems, or organs" *[Stedman's Medical Dictionary]*. Diseases are here categorized according to the repeated appearance of identical symptoms in different patients and summarized into a clinical picture that serves as the benchmark for therapy.

The term **"health"** is defined on the basis of measurable normal values in blood and urine examinations, body temperature, blood pressure, and so on.

In terms of therapeutic concepts, clinical medicine views and treats the patient less as a whole, as a unified system of constant mutually dependent interrelations. Rather, the goal of conventional Western therapy is the particular organ that manifests disturbances or pathological changes. It is for this reason that conventional Western medicine is strictly divided into specialized fields that carry out specifically targeted organ therapies.

Every patient with the same or almost identical clinical picture receives the same organotropically directed medication, in spite of the fact that every one of these patients experiences their disease individually. Patients are hence turned into "cases" for certain diagnostic and medical measures.

Unfortunately, the therapeutic methods of conventional Western medicine thereby quite frequently work against the natural reactions of the organism, that is, blocking and inhibiting the body's power of resistance.

In naturopathic medicine, on the other hand, the terms "**disease**" and "**health**" address the whole person as a unit of complicated interrelationships.

"**Disease**" is defined as the response of the organism's biological defense systems to a prior exogenous or endogenous strain or injury and is—in contrast to the understanding in conventional medicine—regarded as a pathological event that affects the whole person.

Naturopathic medicine understands "**health**" as freedom from various internal and external damages and well-being of the person. **Naturopathic therapies** accord with the natural reactions of the organism and are adjusted to the patient and his or her illness with utmost individuality.

By detoxification and elimination, as well as strengthening and rest, the *biological self-healing mechanisms* of the organism are exclusively supported and stimulated. Thereby they are enabled to control the pathological event with their own strength.

The reason for this is that naturopathic practitioners try to treat with nature, not against it. At the same time, they do not treat the disease, but the patient.

Clinical medicine has so far aimed primarily at treating *acute* and *life-threatening* diseases. Many strong medications that are used today originated at a time when medicine had to fight against acute diseases. Nevertheless, it is very difficult to cure chronic-degenerative diseases, which occur increasingly frequently, with these methods.

Different diseases require different treatment methods.

It is no secret that in spite of the impressive advances of medical science and technology, it is still not always possible to achieve a cure or improvement in many diseases. In such cases, clinical medicine only too frequently likes to turn to palliative remedies with anesthetic or sedative effects.

Some representatives of modern medicine consider therapies with strong effects as the only true treatments against all diseases and impatiently offer the extension of life as justification for these applications, in spite of the fact that everybody knows that it is precisely these treatment methods that frequently disturb the most important barrier against disease, namely the immune system.

As a result, we see an increase in bacteria that are resistant to antibiotics and the return of earlier infectious diseases that were believed to have been defeated.

In addition, chronic-degenerative diseases, malignant growths, allergic hypersensitivities, and intolerances are on the increase.

This situation is further compounded by the effects of toxic pollution in the environment.

The continuous strain on the human body by the consumption of high dosages of chemical medications and additional exposure to environmental toxins poses unnatural demands on the organism that often exceed its capacity for adaptation. This is bound to lead to a weakening and ultimately *blocked regulation* of the immune system, because the human body also has limits in its ability to withstand stress.

Every doctor knows that the human immune system is the most effective weapon against diseases.

Therefore, it is the task of any reasonable therapy not only to treat by fighting diseases with the conventional "canons," but also to secure the preservation of the body's necessary natural stimuli, which strengthen, not weaken, the totality of all vital functions.

It is an extremely positive development that more and more representatives of conventional Western medicine recognize the necessity to take into account the body's own regulatory systems and turn to appropriate supportive therapies.

> **Note**
>
> A constantly growing number of successful therapeutic methods from naturopathic medicine are thereby again incorporated into conventional medicine.

I must stress emphatically at this point that naturopathic medicine cannot replace emergency medicine. Furthermore, nobody denies the valuable achievements in surgery, the successful control of infectious and of acute life-threatening diseases, as well as the achievements of medical technology. On the contrary! These can and must not be replaced by the treatment methods of experiential medicine!

> **Note**
>
> Similarly, it is not disputed that there are diseases in which no naturopathic measures are able to restore health.

Extensive atrophy of β cells in the islets of Langerhans, for example, can often only be counterbalanced by compensatory treatment or substitution therapy.

In cases where no fully functional tissue is left in the hormonal glands, naturopathic methods cannot cause regeneration either.

Nevertheless, in a case of vegetative dysregulation with sluggish functioning in the otherwise intact endocrine tissue, we can obtain better results with naturopathic methods than with substitution since the latter would only further encourage the sluggish glands in their "laziness."

21.3 Why is Cupping Therapy Once Again Indicated in Modern Scientific Medicine at this Particular Time?

Thanks to practitioners of complementary medicine and some physicians, cupping has been preserved through all those years when naturopathic treatment methods were banned from the repertoire of conventional Western medicine. Today, its significance is growing and growing. This is so not only due to its unquestionable efficacy, but also because reputable scientific publications have, especially in the past decades, contributed to research on the cause of the phenomenon of this efficacy.

These therapeutic methods can therefore now also be used by physicians who, up to now, have been exclusively science-oriented. Prerequisites are familiarity with the particularities of cupping and more time for treatment.

> **Note**
>
> Cupping is a healing method that treats without the burden of medications and is absolutely harmless, if applied correctly and appropriately.

This harmlessness of cupping therapy alone is already enough of a recommendation for its application.

In addition, cupping has four decisive advantages:
- First, this therapy largely prevents complications.
- Second, the disease subsides faster.
- Third, resistance is stimulated and remissions therefore occur more rarely.
- And fourth, you can reduce the dosage of chemical medications, as a result of which their negative side-effects are reduced or completely eliminated.

These four points are precisely the reason why cupping therapy is enjoying great popularity with an ever-increasing number of patients! For many of these people, the prospect of cure was hopeless with the methods of clinical medicine or the methods of conventional medicine had failed.

They then experienced for themselves that the gentle therapy of cupping is able to improve or cure many acute, but also painful chronic diseases quickly, safely, and without negative side-effects.

Is this not a further reason for incorporating cupping into the conventional Western treatment methods?

Memorize   **M!**

In many cases, cupping can be used both by itself and as the most logical supplement to necessary clinical measures, in which case its use never disturbs the clinical therapy but only works for the benefit of the patient.

Note

As further comment, I want to note that whenever measures of conventional Western medicine are hopeless, we should never refrain from attempting to apply a naturopathic method that is in accordance with the origin of the disease.

Nobody is allowed to deprive a suffering person of an alleviation of their suffering on the basis of purely emotional dislike or unfounded prejudice!

21.4 Applications of Cupping Therapy in Conventional Medicine

Since I have already reported on the diseases that can be treated by cupping in the practice-oriented Part 3, I will limit myself here to introducing the therapeutic possibilities within clinical medicine.

21.4.1 Acute Diseases

In these types of illness, as for example those of the respiratory paths like **broncho-pneumonia, influenza, pleuritis, and pneumonia,** we can obtain roughly equal results with clinical and with cupping treatment.

For my part, I prefer—with rare exceptions—cupping, and employ, if necessary, homeopathic remedies as supplementary therapy.

Memorize **M!**

In patients with very bad immunity, clinical therapy is preferable.

In these cases, though, cupping stimulates the immune system as supporting therapy and thereby visibly shortens the course of the illness.

In cases where recuperation is slow after the acute manifestations have subsided or, as is often the case, where the patient visits the practitioner only in later stages of the illness, cupping treatment is also very much recommended for fast recovery and prevention of corollary complications.

An example from my clinical practice:

A 28-year-old patient came to my practice with pain during coughing and the diagnosis of "influenza" from two physicians. He had been taking medications for 1 week, which unfortunately had failed to bring relief. Here is what I was able to find out additionally about his illness:

He did not have an elevated temperature.

I placed cups above and below the collar bone as well as on the entire back and on the sides of the thorax region, for a duration of 10 minutes.

Just to be on the safe side, I repeated the treatment after 2 days and prescribed appropriate homeopathic remedies as adjuvant.

There were no complications and the patient regained his health already on the third day.

At the same time, I was able to diagnose his disease as *bronchopneumonia.*

Bronchial asthma can likewise be improved or even cured with repeated cupping, even in apparently hopeless cases. In *purely allergic* bronchial asthma, on the other hand, treatment must include additional therapies like autohemotherapy or autourine therapy besides cupping.

Memorize **M!**

Furthermore, it is important to know that you can quickly end an asthma attack with cupping.

Diseases of the digestive tract, kidneys, and urinary tracts, and cardiovascular disturbances, also all respond well to cupping therapy.

21.4.2 Chronic Diseases

Even chronic diseases with their manifold localizations are a rewarding, if difficult area for cupping treatments.

Unfortunately, in most cases, patients visit naturopathic practitioners only when all other methods have failed. In spite of this, success is visible—even if only after a longer period of time.

For the different forms of **rheumatic disorders,** for example, cupping is suited as **base therapy.** By activating the body's own regulatory mechanisms, it is, of course, not able to make rheumatically changed joints any more supple, but the pain disappears or is at least substantially lessened, and a further progression of the disease is prevented or at least delayed.

In this context, a quote from one of my female patients, directly after cupping on the knee or hip joint: "Immediately after cupping, I always feel like my joints have been oiled."

Persistent pain in the region of the **spinal column, sciatic pain** as **neuritis** or **neuralgia of the sciatic nerve,** and **cervical syndrome** with pain radiating to the back of the head, to the shoulder, and the arms can generally be influenced well with cupping therapy.

As a result of cupping therapy, most patients experience not only alleviation or absence of pain, but also a feeling of relaxation, while there is no strain on the liver or kidneys as well as side-effects like fatigue, which are unavoidable in allopathic pain therapies.

Patients who are being treated with **analgetics** and **antiphlogistics** are able to reduce or even **eliminate** these medications already after short cupping treatment.

For **migraine attacks** with vasoconstriction of the vessels, cupping or cupping massage is the tool of choice. In the vasodilatory stage, however, cupping does not bring any improvement; here, it has diagnostic significance, though, and assists in the fast and correct choice of a remedy or another naturopathic method, for example, neural therapy.

Note

The diagnostic properties of cupping can also be of help to the clinically oriented physician. The reason for this is that there are undefined constellations of symptoms, in which no clinical therapy is truly helpful. In such cases, I advise the application of cupping to still help the patient. At the least, cupping helps to differentiate whether we are dealing with a diseased organ or a vegetative dystonia or even a neurasthenic syndrome. This sounds unbelievable, but only to somebody who has never used cupping.

21.5 Attempting an Evaluation

It would be wrong to focus exclusively on cupping as a matter of principle. Of course we find, as in any healing method, not only opportunities, but also limitations. There are cases in which clinical therapy is absolutely preferable, in which cupping is even bound to fail.

On the other hand, there are diseases in which we can achieve far more with cupping than with conventional treatment methods.

Cupping therapy can initially appear confusing or even frightening to the beginner, especially when it results in a *change for the worse in another part of the body.*

Note

I therefore recommend to begin by collecting experience with respiratory disorders or joint pain, to see how quickly and safely cupping works.

Here, I want to quote Gerhard Bachmann, who wrote the following sentence in his book *Die Schröpfkopfbehandlung* (Cupping Therapy): "It is always striking how patients with pneumonic disorders initially struggle for breath and, stricken by pain, do not dare to breathe deeply, then during cupping treatment breath more quietly and deeply, and often become free of pain after a short time." (Bachmann, 1980) I myself have seen this description confirmed many times.

The incorporation of cupping therapy could considerably enrich clinical medicine, not only because it works quickly and has no negative side-effects, but also because it offers an inexpensive treatment method. This is certainly not insignificant in this age of cost containment in health care.

I believe that cupping therapy is completely risk-free with optimal effectiveness. After 30 years of experience with cupping, both in daily life and in clinical practice, I have never seen it do any harm. The correct application is, of course, indispensable.

Anybody who has employed a combination of clinical medicine and cupping treatment will never want to miss the opportunity again and will be able to select and apply the good and suitable aspects of both areas for the benefit of the patient.

Let me stress emphatically here that cupping does not claim to be the only correct treatment method for all diseases or disease states.

Which method is preferable for a disease is determined on the basis of the clinical picture.

Where would scientific medicine be without experiential medicine? Ultimately, both directions of medicine attempt to restore disturbed health.

We all should finally understand that there is only one medicine. Is it only the treatment methods that differ.

Part 5
Appendix

22 Myths and Facts

Cupping is a treatment method that is particularly susceptible to myths and misinformation. The principle of cupping therapy has remained the same since time immemorial; it is merely that more recently a new technique has been introduced for creating the vacuum in the cup. As a matter of fact, myths about cupping appear again and again that mix fiction with reality and obscure the actual circumstances. This chapter is an attempt to separate out the false information from the facts.

22.1 Myth # 1

There are so-called "vacuum cups" in which the negative pressure is produced by a pump. You often read and learn that the use of these cups is more beneficial because they allow you to create a more intense vacuum, and because they are easier to prime than with the traditional fire cupping technique with glass cups.

Partly true: As a matter of fact, a pump can create such a strong vacuum that the cups will always and in any location on the body suck in the skin and subcutaneous tissue. As a result, the cup is forced to adhere through the mechanical effect.

Even though, with a thermally created vacuum, the glass cups do not always hold the suction or can fall off right after being applied, it must be emphasized that this never happens without reason and is by no means a disadvantage of this cupping technique. The experience of countless generations testifies to this.

As a general rule, it must be noted that a direct comparison between the two cupping techniques would not be objective enough because of the fundamental differences between them in terms of the creation of the vacuum, the basic operating principle, and the cups used.

We must remember a few facts that need to be taken into account in such a comparison:

Both techniques, the relatively recent one with vacuum cups and the traditional, very old one with glass cups, share a common core. Both of them aim to achieve curative effects by means of a vacuum. Both view the removal of disturbances as the therapeutic path to healing. And both have their advantages.

Even though the vacuum in the glass cups is produced by means of heat and cooling air, it is certainly possible to achieve a strong suction. Admittedly, however, a lot of experience is needed in comparison to the use of vacuum cups, where a pump guarantees an intense suction force with very little effort.

With the traditional cupping technique, patients today experience the same effective therapy as that of generations of sick people treated by our medical predecessors. And the fact that fire cupping has been proven effective again and again over such a long time is convincing evidence that the vacuum achieved in this way is sufficient for a successful treatment.

From my perspective, the desire for the cups to achieve suction every time and stay on for the desired length of treatment is certainly understandable. But every practitioner who works with the fire cupping technique knows from experience that a failed vacuum or the immediate falling off of the cups is a useful sign, such as cases of lymph congestion (see knee treatment), severely cramped or hardened muscles, or dry skin areas. For these reasons, the body responds by rejecting the cups and thereby shows the practitioner that a loosening massage, lubrication of the skin, or patience has to be a part of the treatment.

We must note: Whenever practitioners are too fixated on the suctioning of the cups, they will be unable to detect this signal of the body. They must consider the possibility that this might prevent their patients from getting the help they need.

The temptation to force the cups to stay suctioned on is great, especially in beginners. It is, however, a proven fact by now that a stimulus that has a very intense effect on the skin can cause tissue damage. As such, it is certainly possible that existing symptoms can become aggravated if they are treated incorrectly. In cupping therapy, a lesser vacuum often contributes more significantly to the patient's welfare.

Here I do not want to "convert" anybody to the use of either vacuum cups or traditional cupping glasses. Which cupping technique is used should be a decision that is made jointly with the patient.

It might be more beneficial to use the vacuum cups if the patient, or even the practitioner, is afraid of even a small flame.

There are other patients, however, who experience the heat-based suction of glass cups as much more comfortable and effective than the so-called vacuum cups.

To ensure the maximum benefits of a successful cupping therapy for the patient, both cupping techniques have their raison d'etre.

22.2 Myth # 2

Compared with the classical cupping glasses, the application of vacuum cups is more beneficial because it will not cause "undesirable effects" (like burns or formation of thickened, knotted spots or of small blisters).

This is, of course, not true: Burns on the patient during treatment with heated cupping glasses or due to the burning cotton ball are not undesirable effects of the cupping glasses but simply medical malpractice! And this failure in the handling of the flame or the cupping technique is then erroneously equated with undesirable effects.

Likewise, the small lymph-filled blisters are not an undesirable side effect of the cupping glasses. They can form in patients with very sensitive skin. The same holds true for the formation of thickened, knot-like spots in the subcutaneous tissue during cupping, in skinny patients. This is also not a side effect but a situation that occurs very rarely and is related to the patient's constitution. In this type of patient, these manifestations can arise even when we treat them with vacuum cups only.

22.3 Myth # 3

The thinner the cupping glass, the stronger its ability to produce a vacuum and stay suctioned on the skin.

Partly true: Whether the cupping glasses have a thin wall or a thick wall, their suctioning strength is the same. The decisive factor is not the strength of the glass but the volume of each suction cup, which allows it to produce a certain vacuum. Thinner, lighter cups stay on more easily in seated patients. With lying patients, however, the thickness of the glass is irrelevant. I personally only use thick-walled cupping glasses because there is less risk of breakage.

22.4 Myth # 4

When cupping with the traditional cupping technique, the flame should be kept in the cupping glass or below the opening of the glass until the glass is heated up.

Wrong: Heating the cupping glass is a cardinal error!

Memorize	M!

The air in the cupping glass should be warmed up, but without warming or heating the cupping glass itself (see "Cupping Technique," chapter 6)!

Please pay attention that the transition from warming to heating is fluid and that it is very difficult to differentiate between these two processes. This myth likely arose due to ignorance about cupping and about this seemingly simple physical phenomenon. It can, however, result in danger for the patient, and damage the reputation of cupping therapy. As you can see, this myth tasks people who pass on such misinformation about the technique of fire cupping with the responsibility to study cupping with utmost diligence and care.

23 Conclusion

To my delight, interest in cupping therapy has been increasing considerably for the last few years. The fact that scientific studies (Carstens-Stiftung, Natur und Medizin e.V., Presseinformation 2011 and 2012) have now demonstrated for the first time that bleeding cupping in patients with carpal tunnel syndrome and dry cupping in arthrosis of the knee joint lead to a quick and clear alleviation of symptoms is reason enough for me to point to the facts of cupping.

Today, the manifold applications of this method can enrich other therapies and themselves be enriched by different healing methods, including the consumption of chemical medications.

I have attempted to transmit knowledge from the written record, from the experiences of many generations, and from practice about the old healing method of cupping. Cupping is far too valuable of a therapy and must not become discredited yet again as a result of modern myths (as happened in earlier times due to the excessive use of wet cupping).

Continual clinical and research developments will certainly require that one or more of the chapters will need to be supplemented and/or expanded or other diseases added in the future. Nevertheless, I hope for now that I have given the practitioner a sufficiently comprehensive and useful tool for daily practice.

For the student, I hope to have provided inspiration and trust in cupping treatment, and for the patient, I hope to have transmitted interesting information.

24 Figure Credits

Fig. 3.1, 4.3 from Faller A, Schünke M. Der Körper des Menschen. 15th ed. Stuttgart: Thieme; 2008

Fig. 3.2, 4.4, 6.1 from Schünke M, Schulte E, Schumacher U. Prometheus. THIEME Atlas of Anatomy. Head, Neck, and Neuroanatomy. Illustrations by M. Voll and K. Wesker. 3rd ed. Stuttgart: Thieme; 2020

Fig. 4.1 Illustration by Angelika Brauner, Hohenpeißenberg

Fig. 4.2 from Duale Reihe Anatomie. 2nd ed. Stuttgart: Thieme; 2010

Fig. 7.1 © KaWe

All photos: Peter B. Popielski, Bingen, Germany.

25 Bibliography

[1] Abele J. Schröpfkopfbehandlung. 10th ed. Stuttgart: Haug; 2013

[2] Abele J, Herz K. Die Eigenharnbehandlung. 10th ed. Heidelberg: Haug; 1996

[3] Abele J, Das Schröpfen. 5th ed. München: Urban & Fischer in Elsevier; 2005

[4] Armstrong JW. The Water of Life. England: Rupa Paperback; 1944

[5] Aschner B. Technik der Konstitutionstherapie. Heidelberg: Haug; 1949

[6] Assman D. Die Wetterfühligkeit des Menschen. Ursachen und Pathogenese der biologischen Wetterwirkung. Jena: Gustav Fischer; 1955

[7] Bach H-D. Äußere Kennzeichen innerer Erkrankungen. 11th ed. Tutzing: Bio Ritter; 2002

[8] Bachmann G. Die Schröpfkopfbehandlung. Heidelberg: Haug; 1980

[9] Bachmann G. Die Akupunktur eine Ordnungstherapie. Ulm: Haug; 1959

[10] Bässler K-H, Golly I, Loew D, Pietrzik K. Vitamin-Lexikon. 3rd ed. München: Urban & Fischer in Elsevier; 2002

[11] Bayr G. Hahnemanns Selbstversuch mit der Chinarinde im Jahre 1790. Heidelberg: Haug; 1996

[12] Bier A. Hyperämie als Heilmittel. 2nd ed. Leipzig: Verlag von F.C.W. Vogel; 1907

[13] Bischko J. Einführung in die Akupunktur. Heidelberg: Haug; 1972

[14] Boericke W. Homöopathische Mittel und ihre Wirkungen, Materia Medica. 8. Aufl. Leer: Grundlagen und Praxis; 2004

[15] Braun A. Methodik der Homöotherapie. 7th ed. Stuttgart: Sonntag; 2002

[16] Braun H. Heilpflanzen-Lexikon für Ärzte und Apotheker. Stuttgart: Fischer; 1981

[17] Breindl E. Das große Gesundheitsbuch der Hl. Hildegard von Bingen. München: Bassermann; 2004

[18] Brühl W, Brzozowski R. Vademecum Lekarza ogolnego: Warszawa: PZWL; 1990

[19] Claussen C-F. Homotoxikologie. Baden-Baden: Aurelia; 1995

[20] Cornelius A. Die Nervenpunkte. Heidelberg: Haug; 1980

[21] Cornelius P. Nosoden und Begleittherapie. 4th ed. München: Pflaum; 2005

[22] Dorcsi M. Bewährte Indikationen der Homöopathie. Karlsruhe: DHU; 1989

[23] Dosch P. Lehrbuch der Neuraltherapie nach Huneke. 14th ed. Heidelberg: Haug; 1995

[24] Enders N. Bewährte Anwendung der Homöopathischen Arznei. 4th ed. Stuttgart: Haug; 2004

[25] Faller A. Der Körper des Menschen. 15th ed. Stuttgart: Thieme; 2008

[26] Faller A. Anatomie in Stichworten. Stuttgart: Enke; 1980

[27] Forschungsinstitut für chinesische traditionelle Medizin Shanghai. Akupunkturpunkte und Meridiane. Shanghai: Wissenschaft und Technik; 1980

[28] Gaisbauer M. Homöotherapie neurologischer Erkrankungen. Stuttgart: Sonntag; 1993

[29] Gauß F. Wie finde ich das passende Arzneimittel? 9th ed. Heidelberg: Haug; 1996

[30] Gebhardt K-H. Stauffers Homöopathisches Taschenbuch. 27th ed. Stuttgart: Haug; 2004

[31] Haferkamp H. Die Eigenblutbehandlung. Stuttgart: Hippokrates; 1951

[32] Hafter E, Hotz HW, Deucher F. Praktische Gastroenterologie. 7th ed. Stuttgart: Thieme; 1988

[33] Hansen K, von Staa H. Reflektorische und algetische Krankheitszeichen der inneren Organe. Stuttgart: Thieme; 1938

[34] Harrer H. Sieben Jahre in Tibet. 28th ed. Berlin: Ullstein; 2006

[35] Head H. On the disturbances of sensation, with special reference to the pain of visceral disease. Brain, 1893; 16(1-2):1–133

[36] Heilmann K. Arzneimittel der Zukunft. München: Droemersche Verlagsanstalt Th. Knaur Nachf.; 1991

[37] Herzberger G. Grundlagen der Homotoxikologie. 4th ed. Baden-Baden: Aurelia; 1996

[38] Höppe P, von Mackensen S, Nowak D, Piel E. Prävalenz von Wetterfühligkeit in Deutschland. Dtsch Med Wochenschr. 2002; 127(1–2):15–20

[39] Höveler V. Eigenbluttherapie. 7th ed. Heidelberg: Haug; 1998

[40] Hufeland CW. Makrobiotik oder die Kunst, das menschliche Leben zu verlängern. Frankfurt a.M.: Insel; 1984

[41] Illing K-H. Homöopathie für Anfänger. 4th ed. Heidelberg: Haug; 1992

[42] Jablonska S. Choroby Skory. Warszawa: PZWL; 1958

[43] Jovanovic L, Subak-Sharpe N, Genell J. Hormone. München: Heyne; 1991

[44] Julian O. Materia medica der Nosoden. 10th ed. Stuttgart: Haug; 2004

[45] Kent JT. Homöopathische Arzneimittelbilder. 2. Aufl. Stuttgart: Haug; 2009

[46] Kneipp-Heilmittel-Werk. Der Weg zu Kneipp ein Weg zur Gesundheit. Bad Wörishofen: Kneipp Wörisanahaus; 1970

[47] Krauss T. Die Grundgedanken der Iso-Komplex-Heilweise. Stuttgart: Sonntag; 1956

[48] Kuznicka B, Dziak M. Ziola i ich zastosowanie. Warszawa: PZWL; 1987

[49] Lang W. Akupunktur und Nervensystem. 2nd ed. Heidelberg: Haug; 1997

[50] Leibold G. Wetterfühligkeit. Zürich: Oesch; 2000

[51] Lohmann D, Schubert W, Schubert M. Symptome und Diagnostik innerer Krankheiten. 5th ed. Leipzig: Barth; 1994

[52] Marquardt H. Reflexotherapy of the Feet. 2nd ed. Stuttgart: Thieme; 2016

[53] Mességué M. Von Menschen und Pflanzen. Berlin: Ullstein; 2001

[54] Mességué M. Das Mességué Heilkräuterlexikon. Berlin: Ullstein; 2002

[55] Mezger J. Gesichtete Homöopathische Arzneimittellehre. 12th ed. Stuttgart: Haug; 2005

[56] Milka T. Fizykoterapia. Warszawa: PZWL; 1983

[57] Pálos S. Chinesische Ohr-Akupunktur. München: Cedip; 1983

[58] Pischinger A. Das System der Grundregulation. 12th ed. Stuttgart: Haug; 2014

[59] Prusinski A. Podstawy neurologii klinicznej. Warszawa: PZWL; 1983

[60] Pschyrembel, Klinisches Wörterbuch. Berlin: DeGruyter; 1982

[61] Rehm E. Fibel der Homöopathie. Göppingen: Staufen-Pharma; 1973

[62] Scheidt W. Lehrbuch der Neurologie. 5 Aufl. Stuttgart: Thieme; 1980

[63] Schettler G. Innere Medizin. 9th ed. Stuttgart: Thieme; 1997

[64] Schimpfky R. Unsere Heilpflanzen in Bild und Wort. Gera-Untermhaus: Köhler; 1983

[65] Selye H. Streß beherrscht unser Leben. Düsseldorf: Econ; 1957

[66] Sigerist HE. Anfänge der Medizin. Zürich: Europa; 1963

[67] Silbernagl S, Lang F. Color Atlas of Pathophysiology. Stuttgart: Thieme; 2016

[68] Stauffer K. Klinische homöopathische Arzneimittellehre. 14th ed. Stuttgart: Sonntag; 2002

[69] Vermeulen F. Kindertypen in der Homöopathie. 7th ed. Stuttgart: Sonntag; 2007

[70] Wagner F. Reflexzonen-Massage. München: Gräfe & Unzer; 2004

[71] Waldemar C. Großer Akupunktur Bildatlas. Wiesbaden: Englisch; München und Zürich: Perseus; 1900

[72] Wendt L, Wendt T. Angiopathien – Eiweißspeicherkrankheiten – Autoimmunkrankheiten. Heidelberg: Haug; 1980

[73] Wiesenauer M. Gynäkologischgeburtshilfliche Praxis der Homöopathie. 3rd ed. Stuttgart: Hippokrates; 1998

[74] Wiesenauer M. Praxis der Homöopathie. 4th ed. Stuttgart: Hippokrates; 2004

[75] Ziegler H. Vitamine. Hamburg: Germa Press; 1986

Index

Index

Note: Page numbers set **bold** or *italic* indicate headings or figures, respectively.

165